Computational Neuroscience

Computational Neuroscience

Edited by Maurice Abbot

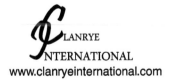

CLANRYE
INTERNATIONAL
www.clanryeinternational.com

Clanrye International,
750 Third Avenue, 9th Floor,
New York, NY 10017, USA

ISBN: 978-1-63240-702-3

Cataloging-in-Publication Data

Computational neuroscience / edited by Maurice Abbot.
    p. cm.
Includes bibliographical references and index.
ISBN 978-1-63240-702-3
1. Computational neuroscience. 2. Nervous system--Computer simulation.
3. Neurosciences--Data processing. I. Abbot, Maurice.
QP357.5 .C66 2018
612.8--dc23

For information on all Clanrye International publications
visit our website at www.clanryeinternational.com

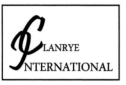

Contents

Preface

Computational neuroscience studies the information processing properties of the different structures present in the human brain. It incorporates the theories like neural networks, computational learning theory and machine learning to study the nervous system. It also uses the elements of psychology, neuroscience, mathematics, cognitive science, etc. to analyze the structures of the nervous system. This textbook is a valuable compilation of topics, ranging from the basic to the most complex theories and principles in the field of computational neuroscience. The topics included in it are of utmost significance and bound to provide incredible insights to readers. It will serve as a valuable source of reference for those interested in this field.

To facilitate a deeper understanding of the contents of this book a short introduction of every chapter is written below:

Chapter 1- Computational neuroscience is an interdisciplinary branch that studies the information processes of the brain in relation to the nervous system. The part of the body that transmits signals and coordinates motor actions is called the nervous system. It is majorly divided into the central nervous system comprising brain and the spinal cord and peripheral nervous system which are composed of nerves. This is an introductory chapter which will introduce briefly all the significant aspects of computational neuroscience.

Chapter 2- The section combines neurons' electrophysiological basis of electrical signaling and its anatomy. The components of neural signaling include signal propagation along the dendrite towards the soma, signal propagation along the axon, spatial and temporal summation in the soma, and neurotransmission across the synapse. The text also focuses on concepts of artificial neuron, FitzHugh–Nagumo model, Morris–Lecar model, etc.

Chapter 3- Artificial neural networks are made up of connected artificial neurons, which carry activation signals. One of the most prominent types of artificial neural network is recurrent neural network. The connection formed through this are in a directed cycle form. The major components of neural networks are discussed in this chapter.

Chapter 4- Unsupervised machine learning ascertains a function to find the hidden data from unlabeled data as opposed to supervised machine learning, which conducts the same operation from labeled data. The section explores the concept of Hebbian theory, which is one of the major approaches taken by unsupervised machine learning. It comes up with an explanation to the adaption of neurons during the learning process. The major forms of unsupervised machine learning are dealt with great details in the section.

I owe the completion of this book to the never-ending support of my family, who supported me throughout the project.

Editor

Understanding Computational Neuroscience

Computational neuroscience is an interdisciplinary branch that studies the information processes of the brain in relation to the nervous system. The part of the body that transmits signals and coordinates motor actions is called the nervous system. It is majorly divided into the central nervous system comprising brain and the spinal cord and peripheral nervous system which are composed of nerves. This is an introductory chapter which will introduce briefly all the significant aspects of computational neuroscience.

Computational Neuroscience

Our understanding of mind and brain has come a long way over the millennia.

There was a time when people did not know that brain is the key organ responsible for our subjective experience. Greek philosopher Aristotle thought that the heart is the "seat of the soul" and the substrate for experience and selfhood. French philosopher Rene Descartes imagined that motor action is possible due to the action of "animal spirits" that rush through the nerves. The history of brain teaches us that though there was a considerable understanding of the brain's structure (anatomy) even half a millennium ago, when it came to brain function, all sorts of fantasies were paraded as knowledge for many centuries.

Around the middle of 18th century, with developments in physics and physiology, a physics- based understanding of brain function began to take shape. It became clear that nerve signals are not "animal spirits" but electric signals not very different from the currents that flow in an electrical circuit. Developments in microscope revealed the peculiar hairy morphology of neurons, and presented a vision of brain as a network of neurons. Progress in neurochemistry, neuropharmacology and neurophysiology unraveled how neurons converse among themselves using chemical signals. Breakthroughs in technology is offering us vast treasures of neuroscientific data spanning many scales from single molecules, to neurons, to networks to whole brain and behavior.

Understanding the brain as an organ is very different from understanding other organs of the body. The brain, first and foremost, is an information processing machine. Like any other organ in the body, the brain too is a mass of cells. But unlike any other organ in the body, brain is a network of cells, a network that clearly distinguishes itself in its sheer size, complexity and lability. An adult brain has about 100 billion neurons, each with about 1,000-10,000 connections. We thus have a staggering figure of about 10^{14}-10^{15} connections in the brain. Therefore, the brain network is perhaps more complex than the entire mobile network of the world, even if we assume that every one of the 7 billion denizens of the planet possess a mobile phone. Furthermore, this extremely complex cerebral network is quite labile, with neurons making and breaking connections at a time-scale that can be as short as a few tens of seconds.

Understanding brain function therefore means the ability to explain brain function in terms of the operations of this complex neural network. Thus the question "how does the brain see?" must be rephrased as "how do networks of neurons in the visual processing areas of the brain transduce the optical image that falls on the retina and process its many properties like form, color, motion etc?" And the answers to these questions are best clothed in the language of mathematics, which is the primary preoccupation of the science of computational neuroscience.

Models of brain can be classified broadly into two types: 1) biophysically realistic models and 2) abstract models. Biophysically realistic models are rooted in biophysics of neuron and brain, and aim to describe brain function in terms of electrical and chemical signaling of the brain. But these models can get extremely complex, computationally challenging, and often offer little insight into the essential information processing mechanisms that govern the function of a neural system. Therefore, modelers constant try to strike a balance between neurobiological realism with reliable and convenient abstraction. The present course also follows a course of development that starts from a biophysically realistic description, tending towards more abstract models by progressive and systematic simplification.

Computational neuroscience (also theoretical neuroscience) studies brain function in terms of the information processing properties of the structures that make up the nervous system. It is an inter-disciplinary computational science that links the diverse fields of neuroscience, cognitive science, and psychology with electrical engineering, computer science, mathematics, and physics.

Computational neuroscience is distinct from psychological connectionism and from learning theories of disciplines such as machine learning, neural networks, and computational learning theory in that it emphasizes descriptions of functional and biologically realistic neurons (and neural systems) and their physiology and dynamics. These models capture the essential features of the biological system at multiple spatial-temporal scales, from membrane currents, proteins, and chemical coupling to network oscillations, columnar and topographic architecture, and learning and memory.

These computational models are used to frame hypotheses that can be directly tested by biological or psychological experiments.

History

The term "computational neuroscience" was introduced by Eric L. Schwartz, who organized a conference, held in 1985 in Carmel, California, at the request of the Systems Development Foundation to provide a summary of the current status of a field which until that point was referred to by a variety of names, such as neural modeling, brain theory and neural networks. The proceedings of this definitional meeting were published in 1990 as the book *Computational Neuroscience*. The first open international meeting focused on Computational Neuroscience was organized by James M. Bower and John Miller in San Francisco, California in 1989 and has continued each year since as the annual CNS meeting. The first graduate educational program in computational neuroscience was organized as the Computational and Neural Systems Ph.D. program at the California Institute of Technology in 1985.

The early historical roots of the field can be traced to the work of people such as Louis Lapicque, Hodgkin & Huxley, Hubel & Wiesel, and David Marr, to name a few. Lapicque introduced the integrate and fire model of the neuron in a seminal article published in 1907; this model is still one of the most popular models in computational neuroscience for both cellular and neural networks studies, as well as in mathematical neuroscience because of its simplicity. About 40 years later, Hodgkin & Huxley developed the voltage clamp and created the first biophysical model of the action potential. Hubel & Wiesel discovered that neurons in the primary visual cortex, the first cortical area to process information coming from the retina, have oriented receptive fields and are organized in columns. David Marr's work focused on the interactions between neurons, suggesting computational approaches to the study of how functional groups of neurons within the hippocampus and neocortex interact, store, process, and transmit information. Computational modeling of biophysically realistic neurons and dendrites began with the work of Wilfrid Rall, with the first multicompartmental model using cable theory.

Major Topics

Research in computational neuroscience can be roughly categorized into several lines of inquiry. Most computational neuroscientists collaborate closely with experimentalists in analyzing novel data and synthesizing new models of biological phenomena.

Single-neuron Modeling

Even single neurons have complex biophysical characteristics and can perform computations (e.g.). Hodgkin and Huxley's original model only employed two voltage-sensitive currents (Voltage sensitive ion channels are glycoprotein molecules which extend through the lipid bilayer, allowing ions to traverse under certain conditions through the axolemma), the fast-acting sodium and the inward-rectifying potassium. Though successful in predicting the timing and qualitative features of the action potential, it nevertheless failed to predict a number of important features such as adaptation and shunting. Scientists now believe that there are a wide variety of voltage-sensitive currents, and the implications of the differing dynamics, modulations, and sensitivity of these currents is an important topic of computational neuroscience.

The computational functions of complex dendrites are also under intense investigation. There is a large body of literature regarding how different currents interact with geometric properties of neurons.

Some models are also tracking biochemical pathways at very small scales such as spines or synaptic clefts.

There are many software packages, such as GENESIS and NEURON, that allow rapid and systematic *in silico* modeling of realistic neurons. Blue Brain, a project founded by Henry Markram from the École Polytechnique Fédérale de Lausanne, aims to construct a biophysically detailed simulation of a cortical column on the Blue Gene supercomputer.

A problem in the field is that detailed neuron descriptions are computationally expensive and this can handicap the pursuit of realistic network investigations, where many neurons need to be simulated. So, researchers that study large neural circuits typically represent each neuron and synapse simply, ignoring much of the biological detail. This is unfortunate as there is evidence that the richness of biophysical properties on the single neuron scale can supply mechanisms that serve as the building blocks for network dynamics. Hence there is a drive to produce simplified neuron models that can retain significant biological fidelity at a low computational overhead. Algorithms have been developed to produce faithful, faster running, simplified surrogate neuron models from computationally expensive, detailed neuron models.

Development, Axonal Patterning, and Guidance

How do axons and dendrites form during development? How do axons know where to target and how to reach these targets? How do neurons migrate to the proper position in the central and peripheral systems? How do synapses form? We know from molecular biology that distinct parts of the nervous system release distinct chemical cues, from growth factors to hormones that modulate and influence the growth and development of functional connections between neurons.

Theoretical investigations into the formation and patterning of synaptic connection and morphology are still nascent. One hypothesis that has recently garnered some attention is the *minimal wiring hypothesis*, which postulates that the formation of axons and dendrites effectively minimizes resource allocation while maintaining maximal information storage.

Sensory Processing

Early models of sensory processing understood within a theoretical framework are credited to Horace Barlow. Somewhat similar to the minimal wiring hypothesis described in the preceding section, Barlow understood the processing of the early sensory systems to be a form of efficient coding, where the neurons encoded information which minimized the number of spikes. Experimental and computational work have since supported this hypothesis in one form or another.

Current research in sensory processing is divided among a biophysical modelling of different subsystems and a more theoretical modelling of perception. Current models of perception have suggested that the brain performs some form of Bayesian inference and integration of different sensory information in generating our perception of the physical world.

Memory and Synaptic Plasticity

Earlier models of memory are primarily based on the postulates of Hebbian learning. Biologically relevant models such as Hopfield net have been developed to address the properties of associative, rather than content-addressable, style of memory that occur in biological systems. These attempts are primarily focusing on the formation of medium- and long-term memory, localizing in the hippocampus. Models of working memory, relying on theories of network oscillations and persistent activity, have been built to capture some features of the prefrontal cortex in context-related memory.

One of the major problems in neurophysiological memory is how it is maintained and changed through multiple time scales. Unstable synapses are easy to train but also prone to stochastic disruption. Stable synapses forget less easily, but they are also harder to consolidate. One recent computational hypothesis involves cascades of plasticity that allow synapses to function at multiple time scales. Stereochemically detailed models of the acetylcholine receptor-based synapse with the Monte Carlo method, working at the time scale of microseconds, have been built. It is likely that computational tools will contribute greatly to our understanding of how synapses function and change in relation to external stimulus in the coming decades.

Behaviors of Networks

Biological neurons are connected to each other in a complex, recurrent fashion. These connections are, unlike most artificial neural networks, sparse and usually specific. It is not known how information is transmitted through such sparsely connected networks. It is also unknown what the computational functions of these specific connectivity patterns are, if any.

The interactions of neurons in a small network can be often reduced to simple models such as the Ising model. The statistical mechanics of such simple systems are well-characterized theoretically. There has been some recent evidence that suggests that dynamics of arbitrary neuronal networks can be reduced to pairwise interactions. It is not known, however, whether such descriptive dynamics impart any important computational function. With the emergence of two-photon microscopy and calcium imaging, we now have powerful experimental methods with which to test the new theories regarding neuronal networks.

In some cases the complex interactions between *inhibitory* and *excitatory* neurons can be simplified using mean field theory, which gives rise to the population model of neural networks. While many neurotheorists prefer such models with reduced complexity, others argue that uncovering structural functional relations depends on including as much neuronal and network structure as possible. Models of this type are typically built in large simulation platforms like GENESIS or NEURON. There have been some attempts to provide unified methods that bridge and integrate these levels of complexity.

Cognition, Discrimination and Learning

Computational modeling of higher cognitive functions has only recently begun. Experimental data comes primarily from single-unit recording in primates. The frontal lobe and parietal lobe function as integrators of information from multiple sensory modalities. There are some tentative ideas regarding how simple mutually inhibitory functional circuits in these areas may carry out biologically relevant computation.

The brain seems to be able to discriminate and adapt particularly well in certain contexts. For instance, human beings seem to have an enormous capacity for memorizing and recognizing faces. One of the key goals of computational neuroscience is to dissect how biological systems carry out these complex computations efficiently and potentially replicate these processes in building intelligent machines.

The brain's large-scale organizational principles are illuminated by many fields, including biology, psychology, and clinical practice. Integrative neuroscience attempts to consolidate these observations through unified descriptive models and databases of behavioral measures and recordings. These are the bases for some quantitative modeling of large-scale brain activity.

The Computational Representational Understanding of Mind (CRUM) is another attempt at modeling human cognition through simulated processes like acquired rule-based systems in decision making and the manipulation of visual representations in decision making.

Consciousness

One of the ultimate goals of psychology/neuroscience is to be able to explain the everyday experience of conscious life. Francis Crick and Christof Koch made some attempts to formulate a consistent framework for future work in neural correlates of consciousness (NCC), though much of the work in this field remains speculative.

Computational Clinical Neuroscience

It is a field that brings together experts in neuroscience, neurology, psychiatry, decision sciences and computational modeling to quantitatively define and investigate problems in neurological and psychiatric diseases, and to train scientists and clinicians that wish to apply these models to diagnosis and treatment.

Notable Persons

- Phil Husbands, professor of computer science and artificial intelligence at the English University of Sussex

- Read Montague, American neuroscientist and popular science author

- Tomaso Poggio, Eugene McDermott professor in the Department of Brain and Cognitive Sciences, investigator at the McGovern Institute for Brain Research, a member of the MIT Computer Science and Artificial Intelligence Laboratory (CSAIL) and director of both the Center for Biological and Computational Learning at MIT and the Center for Brains, Minds, and Machines.

- Terry Sejnowski, investigator at the Howard Hughes Medical Institute and the Francis Crick Professor at The Salk Institute for Biological Studies where he directs the Computational Neurobiology Laboratory

- Haim Sompolinsky, William N. Skirball Professor of Neuroscience at the Edmond and Lily Safra Center for Brain Sciences (formerly the Interdisciplinary Center for Neural Computation), and a Professor of Physics at the Racah Institute of Physics at The Hebrew University of Jerusalem, Israel.

Neuron

A neuron is an electrically excitable cell that processes and transmits information through electrical and chemical signals. These signals between neurons occur via specialized connections called synapses. Neurons can connect to each other to form neural networks. Neurons are major components of the brain and spinal cord of the central nervous system (CNS), and of the autonomic ganglia of the peripheral nervous system.

There are several types of specialized neurons. Sensory neurons respond to stimuli such as touch, sound or light and all other stimuli affecting the cells of the sensory organs that then send signals to the spinal cord and brain. Motor neurons receive signals from the brain and spinal cord to cause muscle contractions and affect glandular outputs. Interneurons connect neurons to other neurons within the same region of the brain, or spinal cord in neural networks.

A typical neuron consists of a cell body (soma), dendrites, and an axon. The term neurite is used to describe either a dendrite or an axon, particularly in its undifferentiated stage. Dendrites are thin structures that arise from the cell body, often extending for hundreds of micrometres and branching multiple times, giving rise to a complex "dendritic tree". An axon (also called a nerve fiber when myelinated) is a special cellular extension (process) that arises from the cell body at a site called the axon hillock and travels for a distance, as far as 1 meter in humans or even more in other species. Nerve fibers are often bundled into fascicles, and in the peripheral nervous system, bundles of fascicles make up nerves (like strands of wire make up cables). The cell body of a neuron frequently gives rise to multiple dendrites, but never to more than one axon, although the axon may branch hundreds of times before it terminates. At the majority of synapses, signals are sent from the axon of one neuron to a dendrite of another. There are, however, many exceptions to these rules: for example, neurons can lack dendrites, or have no axon, and synapses can connect an axon to another axon or a dendrite to another dendrite.

All neurons are electrically excitable, maintaining voltage gradients across their membranes by means of metabolically driven ion pumps, which combine with ion channels embedded in the membrane to generate intracellular-versus-extracellular concentration differences of ions such as sodium, potassium, chloride, and calcium. Changes in the cross-membrane voltage can alter the function of voltage-dependent ion channels. If the voltage changes by a large enough amount, an all-or-none electrochemical pulse called an action potential is generated, which travels rapidly along the cell's axon, and activates synaptic connections with other cells when it arrives.

In most cases, neurons are generated by special types of stem cells. Neurons in the adult brain generally do not undergo cell division. Astrocytes are star-shaped glial cells that have also been observed to turn into neurons by virtue of the stem cell characteristic pluripotency. Neurogenesis largely ceases during adulthood in most areas of the brain. However, there is strong evidence for generation of substantial numbers of new neurons in two brain areas, the hippocampus and olfactory bulb.

Overview

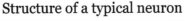

Structure of a typical neuron

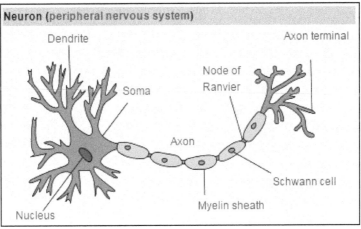

A neuron is a specialized type of cell found in the bodies of all eumetozoans. Only sponges and a few other simpler animals lack neurons. The features that define a neuron are electrical excitability and the presence of synapses, which are complex membrane junctions that transmit signals to other cells. The body's neurons, plus the glial cells that give them structural and metabolic support, together constitute the nervous system. In vertebrates, the majority of neurons belong to the central nervous system, but some reside in peripheral ganglia, and many sensory neurons are situated in sensory organs such as the retina and cochlea.

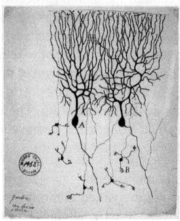

Drawing of neurons in the pigeon cerebellum, by Spanish neuroscientist Santiago Ramón y Cajal in 1899. (A) denotes Purkinje cells and (B) denotes granule cells, both of which are multipolar

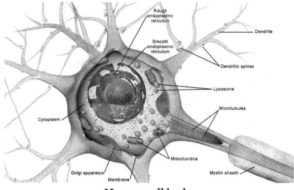

Neuron cell body

A typical neuron is divided into three parts: the soma or cell body, dendrites, and axon. The soma is usually compact; the axon and dendrites are filaments that extrude from it. Dendrites typically branch profusely, getting thinner with each branching, and extending their farthest branches a few hundred micrometers from the soma. The axon leaves the soma at a swelling called the axon hillock, and can extend for great distances, giving rise to hundreds of branches. Unlike dendrites, an axon usually maintains the same diameter as it extends. The soma may give rise to numerous dendrites, but never to more than one axon. Synaptic signals from other neurons are received by the soma and dendrites; signals to other neurons are transmitted by the axon. A typical synapse, then, is a contact between the axon of one neuron and a dendrite or soma of another. Synaptic signals may be excitatory or inhibitory. If the net excitation received by a neuron over a short period of time is large enough, the neuron generates a brief pulse called an action potential, which originates at the soma and propagates rapidly along the axon, activating synapses onto other neurons as it goes.

Many neurons fit the foregoing schema in every respect, but there are also exceptions to most parts of it. There are no neurons that lack a soma, but there are neurons that lack dendrites, and others that lack an axon. Furthermore, in addition to the typical axodendritic and axosomatic synapses, there are axoaxonic (axon-to-axon) and dendrodendritic (dendrite-to-dendrite) synapses.

The key to neural function is the synaptic signaling process, which is partly electrical and partly chemical. The electrical aspect depends on properties of the neuron's membrane. Like all animal cells, the cell body of every neuron is enclosed by a plasma membrane, a bilayer of lipid molecules with many types of protein structures embedded in it. A lipid bilayer is a powerful electrical insulator, but in neurons, many of the protein structures embedded in the membrane are electrically active. These include ion channels that permit electrically charged ions to flow across the membrane, and ion pumps that actively transport ions from one side of the membrane to the other. Most ion channels are permeable only to specific types of ions. Some ion channels are voltage gated, meaning that they can be switched between open and closed states by altering the voltage difference across the membrane. Others are chemically gated, meaning that they can be switched between open and closed states by interactions with chemicals that diffuse through the extracellular fluid. The interactions between ion channels and ion pumps produce a voltage difference across the membrane, typically a bit less than 1/10 of a volt at baseline. This voltage has two functions: first, it provides a power source for an assortment of voltage-dependent protein machinery that is embedded in the membrane; second, it provides a basis for electrical signal transmission between different parts of the membrane.

Neurons communicate by chemical and electrical synapses in a process known as neurotransmission, also called synaptic transmission. The fundamental process that triggers the release of neurotransmitters is the action potential, a propagating electrical signal that is generated by exploiting the electrically excitable membrane of the neuron. This is also known as a wave of depolarization.

Anatomy and Histology

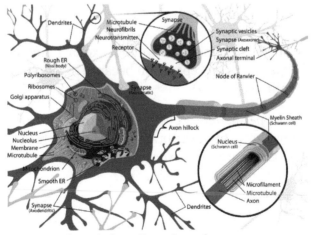

Diagram of a typical myelinated vertebrate motor neuron

Neurons are highly specialized for the processing and transmission of cellular signals. Given their diversity of functions performed in different parts of the nervous system, there is, as expected, a wide variety in their shape, size, and electrochemical properties. For instance, the soma of a neuron can vary from 4 to 100 micrometers in diameter.

- The soma is the body of the neuron. As it contains the nucleus, most protein synthesis occurs here. The nucleus can range from 3 to 18 micrometers in diameter.

- The dendrites of a neuron are cellular extensions with many branches. This overall shape and structure is referred to metaphorically as a dendritic tree. This is where the majority of input to the neuron occurs via the dendritic spine.

- The axon is a finer, cable-like projection that can extend tens, hundreds, or even tens of thousands of times the diameter of the soma in length. The axon carries nerve signals away from the soma (and also carries some types of information back to it). Many neurons have only one axon, but this axon may—and usually will—undergo extensive branching, enabling communication with many target cells. The part of the axon where it emerges from the soma is called the axon hillock. Besides being an anatomical structure, the axon hillock is also the part of the neuron that has the greatest density of voltage-dependent sodium channels. This makes it the most easily excited part of the neuron and the spike initiation zone for the axon: in electrophysiological terms it has the most negative action potential threshold. While the axon and axon hillock are generally involved in information outflow, this region can also receive input from other neurons.

- The axon terminal contains synapses, specialized structures where neurotransmitter chemicals are released to communicate with target neurons.

The canonical view of the neuron attributes dedicated functions to its various anatomical components; however dendrites and axons often act in ways contrary to their so-called main function.

Axons and dendrites in the central nervous system are typically only about one micrometer thick, while some in the peripheral nervous system are much thicker. The soma is usually about 10–25 micrometers in diameter and often is not much larger than the cell nucleus it contains. The longest axon of a human motor neuron can be over a meter long, reaching from the base of the spine to the toes.

Sensory neurons can have axons that run from the toes to the posterior column of the spinal cord, over 1.5 meters in adults. Giraffes have single axons several meters in length running along the entire length of their necks. Much of what is known about axonal function comes from studying the squid giant axon, an ideal experimental preparation because of its relatively immense size (0.5–1 millimeters thick, several centimeters long).

Fully differentiated neurons are permanently postmitotic; however, research starting around 2002 shows that additional neurons throughout the brain can originate from neural stem cells through the process of neurogenesis. These are found throughout the brain, but are particularly concentrated in the subventricular zone and subgranular zone.

Histology and Internal Structure

Numerous microscopic clumps called Nissl substance (or Nissl bodies) are seen when nerve cell bodies are stained with a basophilic ("base-loving") dye. These structures consist of rough endoplasmic reticulum and associated ribosomal RNA. Named after German psychiatrist and neuropathologist Franz Nissl (1860–1919), they are involved in protein synthesis and their prominence can be explained by the fact that nerve cells are very metabolically active. Basophilic dyes such as aniline or (weakly) haematoxylin highlight negatively charged components, and so bind to the phosphate backbone of the ribosomal RNA.

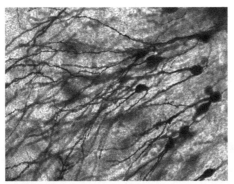

Golgi-stained neurons in human hippocampal tissue

The cell body of a neuron is supported by a complex mesh of structural proteins called neurofilaments, which are assembled into larger neurofibrils. Some neurons also contain pigment granules, such as neuromelanin (a brownish-black pigment that is byproduct of synthesis of catecholamines), and lipofuscin (a yellowish-brown pigment), both of which accumulate with age. Other structural proteins that are important for neuronal function are actin and the tubulin of microtubules. Actin is predominately found at the tips of axons and dendrites during neuronal development.

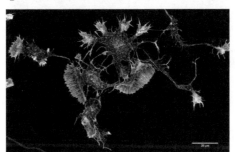

Actin filaments in a mouse Cortical Neuron in culture

There are different internal structural characteristics between axons and dendrites. Typical axons almost never contain ribosomes, except some in the initial segment. Dendrites contain granular endoplasmic reticulum or ribosomes, in diminishing amounts as the distance from the cell body increases.

Classification

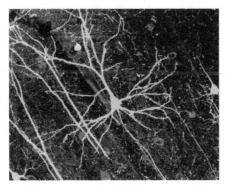

Image of pyramidal neurons in mouse cerebral cortex expressing green fluorescent protein.
The red staining indicates GABAergic interneurons

Neurons exist in a number of different shapes and sizes and can be classified by their morphology and function. The anatomist Camillo Golgi grouped neurons into two types; type I with long axons used to move signals over long distances and type II with short axons, which can often be confused with dendrites. Type I cells can be further divided by where the cell body or soma is located. The basic morphology of type I neurons, represented by spinal motor neurons, consists of a cell body called the soma and a long thin axon covered by the myelin sheath. Around the cell body is a branching dendritic tree that receives signals from other neurons. The end of the axon has branching terminals (axon terminal) that release neurotransmitters into a gap called the synaptic cleft between the terminals and the dendrites of the next neuron.

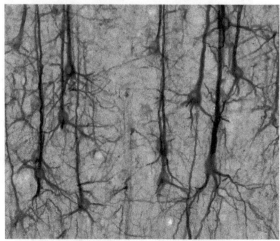

SMI32-stained pyramidal neurons in cerebral cortex

Structural Classification

Polarity

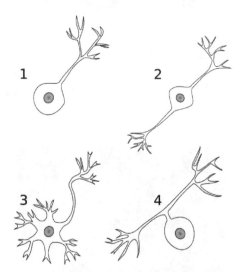

Different kinds of neurons:
1 Unipolar neuron
2 Bipolar neuron
3 Multipolar neuron
4 Pseudounipolar neuron

Most neurons can be anatomically characterized as:

- Unipolar or pseudounipolar: dendrite and axon emerging from same process.

- Bipolar: axon and single dendrite on opposite ends of the soma.

- Multipolar: two or more dendrites, separate from the axon:

  - Golgi I: neurons with long-projecting axonal processes; examples are pyramidal cells, Purkinje cells, and anterior horn cells.

  - Golgi II: neurons whose axonal process projects locally; the best example is the granule cell.

- Anaxonic: where axon cannot be distinguished from dendrites.

Other

Furthermore, some unique neuronal types can be identified according to their location in the nervous system and distinct shape. Some examples are:

- Basket cells, interneurons that form a dense plexus of terminals around the soma of target cells, found in the cortex and cerebellum.

- Betz cells, large motor neurons.

- Lugaro cells, interneurons of the cerebellum.

- Medium spiny neurons, most neurons in the corpus striatum.

- Purkinje cells, huge neurons in the cerebellum, a type of Golgi I multipolar neuron.

- Pyramidal cells, neurons with triangular soma, a type of Golgi I.

- Renshaw cells, neurons with both ends linked to alpha motor neurons.

- Unipolar brush cells, interneurons with unique dendrite ending in a brush-like tuft.

- Granule cells, a type of Golgi II neuron.

- Anterior horn cells, motoneurons located in the spinal cord.

- Spindle cells, interneurons that connect widely separated areas of the brain

Functional Classification

Direction

- Afferent neurons convey information from tissues and organs into the central nervous system and are also called sensory neurons.

- Efferent neurons transmit signals from the central nervous system to the effector cells and are also called motor neurons.

- Interneurons connect neurons within specific regions of the central nervous system.

Afferent and efferent also refer generally to neurons that, respectively, bring information to or send information from the brain.

Action on Other Neurons

A neuron affects other neurons by releasing a neurotransmitter that binds to chemical receptors. The effect upon the postsynaptic neuron is determined not by the presynaptic neuron or by the neurotransmitter, but by the type of receptor that is activated. A neurotransmitter can be thought of as a key, and a receptor as a lock: the same type of key can here be used to open many different types of locks. Receptors can be classified broadly as *excitatory* (causing an increase in firing rate), *inhibitory* (causing a decrease in firing rate), or *modulatory* (causing long-lasting effects not directly related to firing rate).

The two most common neurotransmitters in the brain, glutamate and GABA, have actions that are largely consistent. Glutamate acts on several different types of receptors, and have effects that are excitatory at ionotropic receptors and a modulatory effect at metabotropic receptors. Similarly GABA acts on several different types of receptors, but all of them have effects (in adult animals, at least) that are inhibitory. Because of this consistency, it is common for neuroscientists to simplify the terminology by referring to cells that release glutamate as "excitatory neurons", and cells that release GABA as "inhibitory neurons". Since over 90% of the neurons in the brain release either glutamate or GABA, these labels encompass the great majority of neurons. There are also other types of neurons that have consistent effects on their targets, for example "excitatory" motor neurons in the spinal cord that release acetylcholine, and "inhibitory" spinal neurons that release glycine.

The distinction between excitatory and inhibitory neurotransmitters is not absolute, however. Rather, it depends on the class of chemical receptors present on the postsynaptic neuron. In principle, a single neuron, releasing a single neurotransmitter, can have excitatory effects on some targets, inhibitory effects on others, and modulatory effects on others still. For example, photoreceptor cells in the retina constantly release the neurotransmitter glutamate in the absence of light. So-called OFF bipolar cells are, like most neurons, excited by the released glutamate. However, neighboring target neurons called ON bipolar cells are instead *inhibited* by glutamate, because they lack the typical ionotropic glutamate receptors and instead express a class of inhibitory metabotropic glutamate receptors. When light is present, the photoreceptors cease releasing glutamate, which relieves the ON bipolar cells from inhibition, activating them; this simultaneously removes the excitation from the OFF bipolar cells, silencing them.

It is possible to identify the type of inhibitory effect a presynaptic neuron will have on a postsynaptic neuron, based on the proteins the presynaptic neuron expresses. Parvalbumin-expressing neurons typically dampen the output signal of the postsynaptic neuron in the visual cortex, whereas somatostatin-expressing neurons typically block dendritic inputs to the postsynaptic neuron.

Discharge Patterns

Neurons have intrinsic electroresponsive properties like intrinsic transmembrane voltage oscillatory patterns. So neurons can be classified according to their electrophysiological characteristics:

- Tonic or regular spiking. Some neurons are typically constantly (or tonically) active. Example: interneurons in neurostriatum.

- Phasic or bursting. Neurons that fire in bursts are called phasic.

- Fast spiking. Some neurons are notable for their high firing rates, for example some types of cortical inhibitory interneurons, cells in globus pallidus, retinal ganglion cells.

Classification by Neurotransmitter Production

- Cholinergic neurons—acetylcholine. Acetylcholine is released from presynaptic neurons into the synaptic cleft. It acts as a ligand for both ligand-gated ion channels and metabotropic (GPCRs) muscarinic receptors. Nicotinic receptors, are pentameric ligand-gated ion channels composed of alpha and beta subunits that bind nicotine. Ligand binding opens the channel causing influx of Na^+ depolarization and increases the probability of presynaptic neurotransmitter release. Acetylcholine is synthesized from choline and acetyl coenzyme A.

- GABAergic neurons—gamma aminobutyric acid. GABA is one of two neuroinhibitors in the CNS, the other being Glycine. GABA has a homologous function to ACh, gating anion channels that allow Cl^- ions to enter the post synaptic neuron. Cl^- causes hyperpolarization within the neuron, decreasing the probability of an action potential firing as the voltage becomes more negative (recall that for an action potential to fire, a positive voltage threshold must be reached). GABA is synthesized from glutamate neurotransmitters by the enzyme glutamate decarboxylase.

- Glutamatergic neurons—glutamate. Glutamate is one of two primary excitatory amino acid neurotransmitter, the other being Aspartate. Glutamate receptors are one of four categories, three of which are ligand-gated ion channels and one of which is a G-protein coupled receptor (often referred to as GPCR).

  1. AMPA and Kainate receptors both function as cation channels permeable to Na^+ cation channels mediating fast excitatory synaptic transmission

  2. NMDA receptors are another cation channel that is more permeable to Ca^{2+}. The function of NMDA receptors is dependant on Glycine receptor binding as a co-agonist within the channel pore. NMDA receptors do not function without both ligands present.

  3. Metabotropic receptors, GPCRs modulate synaptic transmission and postsynaptic excitability.

Glutamate can cause excitotoxicity when blood flow to the brain is interrupted, resulting in brain damage. When blood flow is suppressed, glutamate is released from presynaptic neurons causing NMDA and AMPA receptor activation more so than would normally be the case outside of stress conditions, leading to elevated Ca^{2+} and Na^+ entering the post synaptic neuron and cell damage. Glutamate is synthesized from the amino acid glutamine by the enzyme glutamate synthase.

- Dopaminergic neurons—dopamine. Dopamine is a neurotransmitter that acts on D1 type (D1 and D5) Gs coupled receptors, which increase cAMP and PKA, and D2 type (D2, D3, and D4) receptors, which activate Gi-coupled receptors that decrease cAMP and PKA. Dopamine is connected to mood and behavior, and modulates both pre and post synaptic neurotransmission. Loss of dopamine neurons in the substantia nigra has been linked to Parkinson's disease. Dopamine is synthesized from the amino acid tyrosine. Tyrosine is catalyzed into levadopa (or L-DOPA) by tyrosine hydroxlase, and levadopa is then converted into dopamine by amino acid decarboxylase.

- Serotonergic neurons—serotonin. Serotonin (5-Hydroxytryptamine, 5-HT) can act as excitatory or inhibitory. Of the four 5-HT receptor classes, 3 are GPCR and 1 is ligand gated cation channel. Serotonin is synthesized from tryptophan by tryptophan hydroxylase, and then further by aromatic acid decarboxylase. A lack of 5-HT at postsynaptic neurons has been linked to depression. Drugs that block the presynaptic serotonin transporter are used for treatment, such as Prozac and Zoloft.

Connectivity

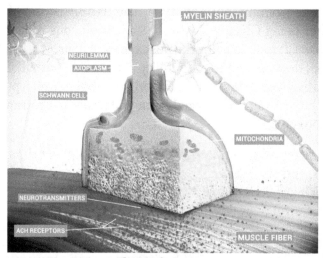

Chemical synapse

Neurons communicate with one another via synapses, where the axon terminal or *en passant* bouton (a type of terminals located along the length of the axon) of one cell contacts another neuron's dendrite, soma or, less commonly, axon. Neurons such as Purkinje cells in the cerebellum can have over 1000 dendritic branches, making connections with tens of thousands of other cells; other neurons, such as the magnocellular neurons of the supraoptic nucleus, have only one or two dendrites, each of which receives thousands of synapses. Synapses can be excitatory or inhibitory and either increase or decrease activity in the target neuron, respectively. Some neurons also communicate via electrical synapses, which are direct, electrically conductive junctions between cells.

In a chemical synapse, the process of synaptic transmission is as follows: when an action potential reaches the axon terminal, it opens voltage-gated calcium channels, allowing calcium ions to enter the terminal. Calcium causes synaptic vesicles filled with neurotransmitter molecules to fuse with the membrane, releasing their contents into the synaptic cleft. The neurotransmitters diffuse across the synaptic cleft and activate receptors on the postsynaptic neuron. High cytosolic calcium in the axon terminal also triggers mitochondrial calcium uptake, which, in turn, activates mitochondrial energy metabolism to produce ATP to support continuous neurotransmission.

The human brain has a huge number of synapses. Each of the 10^{11} (one hundred billion) neurons has on average 7,000 synaptic connections to other neurons. It has been estimated that the brain of a three-year-old child has about 10^{15} synapses (1 quadrillion). This number declines with age, stabilizing by adulthood. Estimates vary for an adult, ranging from 10^{14} to 5×10^{14} synapses (100 to 500 trillion).

Mechanisms for Propagating Action Potentials

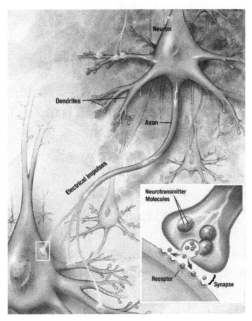

A signal propagating down an axon to the cell body and dendrites of the next cell

In 1937, John Zachary Young suggested that the squid giant axon could be used to study neuronal electrical properties. Being larger than but similar in nature to human neurons, squid cells were easier to study. By inserting electrodes into the giant squid axons, accurate measurements were made of the membrane potential.

The cell membrane of the axon and soma contain voltage-gated ion channels that allow the neuron to generate and propagate an electrical signal (an action potential). These signals are generated and propagated by charge-carrying ions including sodium (Na^+), potassium (K^+), chloride (Cl^-), and calcium (Ca^{2+}).

There are several stimuli that can activate a neuron leading to electrical activity, including pressure, stretch, chemical transmitters, and changes of the electric potential across the cell membrane. Stimuli cause specific ion-channels within the cell membrane to open, leading to a flow of ions through the cell membrane, changing the membrane potential.

Thin neurons and axons require less metabolic expense to produce and carry action potentials, but thicker axons convey impulses more rapidly. To minimize metabolic expense while maintaining rapid conduction, many neurons have insulating sheaths of myelin around their axons. The sheaths are formed by glial cells: oligodendrocytes in the central nervous system and Schwann cells in the peripheral nervous system. The sheath enables action potentials to travel faster than in unmyelinated axons of the same diameter, whilst using less energy. The myelin sheath in peripheral nerves normally runs along the axon in sections about 1 mm long, punctuated by unsheathed nodes of Ranvier, which contain a high density of voltage-gated ion channels. Multiple sclerosis is a neurological disorder that results from demyelination of axons in the central nervous system.

Some neurons do not generate action potentials, but instead generate a graded electrical signal, which in turn causes graded neurotransmitter release. Such nonspiking neurons tend to be sensory neurons or interneurons, because they cannot carry signals long distances.

Neural Coding

Neural coding is concerned with how sensory and other information is represented in the brain by neurons. The main goal of studying neural coding is to characterize the relationship between the stimulus and the individual or ensemble neuronal responses, and the relationships amongst the electrical activities of the neurons within the ensemble. It is thought that neurons can encode both digital and analog information.

All-or-none Principle

The conduction of nerve impulses is an example of an all-or-none response. In other words, if a neuron responds at all, then it must respond completely. Greater intensity of stimulation does not produce a stronger signal but can produce a higher frequency of firing. There are different types of receptor response to stimulus, slowly adapting or tonic receptors respond to steady stimulus and produce a steady rate of firing. These tonic receptors most often respond to increased intensity of stimulus by increasing their firing frequency, usually as a power function of stimulus plotted against impulses per second. This can be likened to an intrinsic property of light where to get greater intensity of a specific frequency (color) there have to be more photons, as the photons can't become "stronger" for a specific frequency.

There are a number of other receptor types that are called quickly adapting or phasic receptors, where firing decreases or stops with steady stimulus; examples include: skin when touched by an object causes the neurons to fire, but if the object maintains even pressure against the skin, the neurons stop firing. The neurons of the skin and muscles that are responsive to pressure and vibration have filtering accessory structures that aid their function.

The pacinian corpuscle is one such structure. It has concentric layers like an onion, which form around the axon terminal. When pressure is applied and the corpuscle is deformed, mechanical stimulus is transferred to the axon, which fires. If the pressure is steady, there is no more stimulus; thus, typically these neurons respond with a transient depolarization during the initial deformation and again when the pressure is removed, which causes the corpuscle to change shape again. Other types of adaptation are important in extending the function of a number of other neurons.

History

The neuron's place as the primary functional unit of the nervous system was first recognized in the late 19th century through the work of the Spanish anatomist Santiago Ramón y Cajal.

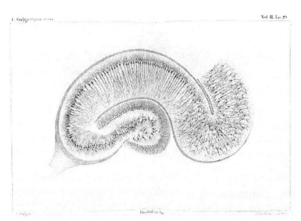

Drawing by Camillo Golgi of a hippocampus stained using the silver nitrate method

To make the structure of individual neurons visible, Ramón y Cajal improved a silver staining process that had been developed by Camillo Golgi. The improved process involves a technique called "double impregnation" and is still in use today.

In 1888 Ramón y Cajal published a paper about the bird cerebellum. In this paper he tells he could not find evidence for anastomis between axons and dendrites and calls each nervous element "an absolutely autonomous canton" This became known as the neuron doctrine, one of the central tenets of modern neuroscience.

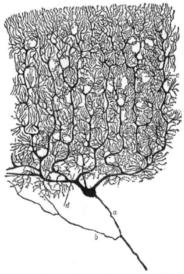

Drawing of a Purkinje cell in the cerebellar cortex done by Santiago Ramón y Cajal, demonstrating the ability of Golgi's staining method to reveal fine detail

In 1891 the German anatomist Heinrich Wilhelm Waldeyer wrote a highly influential review about the neuron doctrine in which he introduced the term *neuron* to describe the anatomical and physiological unit of the nervous system.

The silver impregnation stains are an extremely useful method for neuroanatomical investigations because, for reasons unknown, it stains a very small percentage of cells in a tissue, so one is able to see the complete micro structure of individual neurons without much overlap from other cells in the densely packed brain.

Neuron Doctrine

The neuron doctrine is the now fundamental idea that neurons are the basic structural and functional units of the nervous system. The theory was put forward by Santiago Ramón y Cajal in the late 19th century. It held that neurons are discrete cells (not connected in a meshwork), acting as metabolically distinct units.

Later discoveries yielded a few refinements to the simplest form of the doctrine. For example, glial cells, which are not considered neurons, play an essential role in information processing. Also, electrical synapses are more common than previously thought, meaning that there are direct, cytoplasmic connections between neurons. In fact, there are examples of neurons forming even tighter coupling: the squid giant axon arises from the fusion of multiple axons.

Ramón y Cajal also postulated the Law of Dynamic Polarization, which states that a neuron receives signals at its dendrites and cell body and transmits them, as action potentials, along the axon in one direction: away from the cell body. The Law of Dynamic Polarization has important exceptions; dendrites can serve as synaptic output sites of neurons and axons can receive synaptic inputs.

Neurons in the Brain

The number of neurons in the brain varies dramatically from species to species. The adult human brain contains about 85-86 billion neurons, of which 16.3 billion are in the cerebral cortex and 69 billion in the cerebellum. By contrast, the nematode worm *Caenorhabditis elegans* has just 302 neurons, making it an ideal experimental subject as scientists have been able to map all of the organism's neurons. The fruit fly *Drosophila melanogaster*, a common subject in biological experiments, has around 100,000 neurons and exhibits many complex behaviors. Many properties of neurons, from the type of neurotransmitters used to ion channel composition, are maintained across species, allowing scientists to study processes occurring in more complex organisms in much simpler experimental systems.

Neurological Disorders

Charcot–Marie–Tooth disease (CMT) is a heterogeneous inherited disorder of nerves (neuropathy) that is characterized by loss of muscle tissue and touch sensation, predominantly in the feet and legs but also in the hands and arms in the advanced stages of disease. Presently incurable, this disease is one of the most common inherited neurological disorders, with 37 in 100,000 affected.

Alzheimer's disease (AD), also known simply as Alzheimer's, is a neurodegenerative disease characterized by progressive cognitive deterioration together with declining activities of daily living and neuropsychiatric symptoms or behavioral changes. The most striking early symptom is loss of short-term memory (amnesia), which usually manifests as minor forgetfulness that becomes steadily more pronounced with illness progression, with relative preservation of older memories. As the disorder progresses, cognitive (intellectual) impairment extends to the domains of language (aphasia), skilled movements (apraxia), and recognition (agnosia), and functions such as decision-making and planning become impaired.

Parkinson's disease (PD), also known as Parkinson disease, is a degenerative disorder of the central nervous system that often impairs the sufferer's motor skills and speech. Parkinson's disease belongs to a group of conditions called movement disorders. It is characterized by muscle rigidity, tremor, a slowing of physical movement (bradykinesia), and in extreme cases, a loss of physical movement (akinesia). The primary symptoms are the results of decreased stimulation of the motor cortex by the basal ganglia, normally caused by the insufficient formation and action of dopamine, which is produced in the dopaminergic neurons of the brain. Secondary symptoms may include high level cognitive dysfunction and subtle language problems. PD is both chronic and progressive.

Myasthenia gravis is a neuromuscular disease leading to fluctuating muscle weakness and fatigability during simple activities. Weakness is typically caused by circulating antibodies that block acetylcholine receptors at the post-synaptic neuromuscular junction, inhibiting the stimulative effect of the neurotransmitter acetylcholine. Myasthenia is treated with immunosuppressants, cholinesterase inhibitors and, in selected cases, thymectomy.

Demyelination

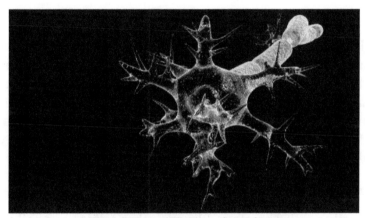

Guillain–Barré syndrome – demyelination

Demyelination is the act of demyelinating, or the loss of the myelin sheath insulating the nerves. When myelin degrades, conduction of signals along the nerve can be impaired or lost, and the nerve eventually withers. This leads to certain neurodegenerative disorders like multiple sclerosis and chronic inflammatory demyelinating polyneuropathy.

Axonal Degeneration

Although most injury responses include a calcium influx signaling to promote resealing of severed parts, axonal injuries initially lead to acute axonal degeneration, which is rapid separation of the proximal and distal ends within 30 minutes of injury. Degeneration follows with swelling of the axolemma, and eventually leads to bead like formation. Granular disintegration of the axonal cytoskeleton and inner organelles occurs after axolemma degradation. Early changes include accumulation of mitochondria in the paranodal regions at the site of injury. Endoplasmic reticulum degrades and mitochondria swell up and eventually disintegrate. The disintegration is dependent on ubiquitin and calpain proteases (caused by influx of calcium ion), suggesting that axonal degeneration is an active process. Thus the axon undergoes complete fragmentation. The process takes about roughly 24 hrs in the PNS, and longer in the CNS. The signaling pathways leading to axolemma degeneration are currently unknown.

Neurogenesis

It has been demonstrated that neurogenesis can sometimes occur in the adult vertebrate brain, a finding that led to controversy in 1999. Later studies of the age of human neurons suggest that this process occurs only for a minority of cells, and a vast majority of neurons comprising the neocortex were formed before birth and persist without replacement.

The body contains a variety of stem cell types that have the capacity to differentiate into neurons. A report in *Nature* suggested that researchers had found a way to transform human skin cells into working nerve cells using a process called transdifferentiation in which "cells are forced to adopt new identities".

Nerve Regeneration

It is often possible for peripheral axons to regrow if they are severed.

Neuron: Structure and Function

In this section, we give a brief outline of the structure and function of a neuron. At the outset, we must note that a neuron is not a specific cell, but a general term given to a large class of cells that share certain properties. This family of cells vary greatly in their morphology and the mechanisms and molecules they use to signal to each other. Therefore, it is impossible to describe the structure and function of neurons in all their rich variety. The description of the structure and function of a typical neuron. The following chapter describes how the processes described verbally in the present chapter may be described mathematically.

Structure of a Neuron

- A neuron is primarily a cell. Therefore, like any other cell it has a cell body wrapped inside a cell membrane. It has a nucleus that contains the chromosomes which constitute the genetic information. It has other standard cellular components, the organelles like mitochondria, golgi bodies, nissil bodies, endoplasmic reticulum and so on. But what distinguishes a neuron from most other cells is the rich and elaborate wiring that seems to emerge from the cell body, also called soma. Neurons vary greatly in terms of the number of these wiry structures that stick out of the cell body. While a neuron like the bipolar cell, found in the retina of the eye, has only two wires sticking out of the soma, there are neurons like the purkinje cell in the cerebellum, which have about one or two lakh wires per cell. In fact, even at a first glance, this wiring seems to be something odd about a neuron. One would not be totally off track if one surmised that it is these wires that make neuron a special cell, and, by extension, the brain a special organ. Hence broadly, depending on the Dendrite, we can classify the Neuron as:

    1) Unipolar cell: 1 wire sticking out of the soma.

    2) Bipolar cell: 2 wires sticking out of the soma.

    3) Multipolar cell: Many wires sticking out of the soma.

    4) Pseudounipolar Neuron.

Structure of a Typical Neuron

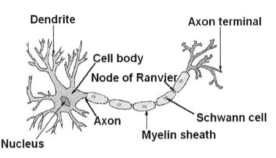

Structure of a neuron

On a closer look, one can distinguish two distinct portions in the wiring system: one portion has shorter, more densely distributed wiring, known as the dendrites; the other portion, consisting typically of a single long wire, known as an axon, branches out into smaller axon terminals at the far end. Neurons use these dendrites and axons to receive and transmit signals to each other. Signals from other neurons are received by the dendrites, while signals to other neurons are transmitted by axon and its terminals. Thus a neuron can be regarded as an input-output system with dendrites as the inputs and the axon terminals as its outputs. Signals from one neuron to another are transmitted across a small gap – between the axon terminal of one neuron and the dendrite of another neuron – known as the synapse.

Electrophysiology of a Neuron

The basis of electrical signaling in a neuron is the fact that there is voltage difference between the interior of the neuron relative to the space surrounding the neuron, the extracellular space. This voltage, known as the membrane potential, is a constant (of about -70 mV) in resting conditions. However, when a neuron is stimulated, by one of several factors, the membrane voltage can show both positive and negative deviations. These voltage variations carry signals across the body of a neuron, and also contribute to signals that are transmitted from one neuron to another across the synapse.

Electrophysiology is a branch of physiology that deals with electrical phenomena related to biological systems. This field of science, in turn, has its roots in electrochemistry, a branch of chemistry that deals with the relationship between ions and electricity, a common example of which is a battery. A basic principle of electrochemistry states that when two compartments containing of an ion X, in different concentrations, are separated by a membrane that is selectively permeable to that ion, then, at equilibrium, voltage difference is generated between the two compartments. This voltage difference, known as the Nernst potential, depends on the ratio of equilibrium ion concentrations in the two compartments.

Ions and Ion Channels

Membrane potential in a neuron, or to that matter in any cell that has a membrane potential, is generated due to a difference in concentrations between the interior of the cell and the extracellular space. There is not one but several ions that contribute to the membrane potential, the key players being: Na+, K+, Cl- and Ca2+. The membrane potential is some sense, a combined effect, of the Nernst potentials of these individual ionic species. But to generate a Nernst potential we mentioned above that we require a semi-permeable membrane. That is to generate a Nernst potential for Na+, we need the membrane to be semi- or selectively permeable to Na+, and so on. What about the membrane produces this semi-permeability or selective permeability?

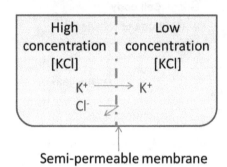

Semi-permeable membrane

Neural Signaling with a semipermeable membrane

Neural membrane is impregnated with tiny pores, known as ion channels, that allow passage of ions. These channels, which are constituted by membrane spanning proteins, are usually selective to specific types of ions. Thus a sodium channel shows high selectivity to Na+ ions, though it allows passage of minute quantities of other ions. Similar is the case with channels of other ions – potassium channels, chloride channels, calcium channels etc.

Different ions are distributed differently across the neural membrane. For example, in resting conditions, sodium concentration is higher outside the cell, than inside. Therefore the Nernst potential of sodium is positive inside. Thus when only sodium ions are present, the membrane potential is equal to the Nernst potential of sodium, i.e., positive inside. On the contrary, potassium ion concentration is higher within the cell than without, making the corresponding Nernst potential negative inside. Thus when only potassium ions are present, Nernst potential is negative inside.

$$V_1 - V_2 = \frac{RT}{Z_x F} \ln \frac{[X]_2}{[X]_1}$$

V1 – V2 = nernst potential for ion 'X'

$[X]_{1,2}$ = concentrations of 'X'

Z_x = Valence of 'X'

T = Absolute temperature

F = Faradays' constant

$RT/F = 26\,mV$ at $T = 25°C\{Z_x = \pm1\}$

The ability of a channel.to allow ions is not fixed for all time. Channels can be in OPEN or CLOSED states. A channel in OPEN state has naturally greater permeability than in CLOSED state. OPEN channels. Also offer greater electrical conductance to the ions to which they are permeable.

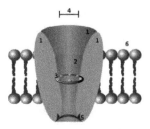

- **1** - channel domains(typically four per channel),
- **2** - outer vestibule,
- **3** - selectivity filter,
- **4** - diameter of selectivity filter,
- **5** - phosphorylation site, **6** - cell membrane.

Structure of a Channel

The conductance of a channel determines the contribution of the Nernst potential of the corresponding ionic species, to the membrane potential. Earlier we stated that, when only potassium ions are present, the membrane potential is negative, and when only sodium ions are present, the membrane potential is positive. Now we consider a small variation of that scenario. Consider a situation when both sodium and potassium ions are present (with the usual intra- and extra-cellular distributions) but only potassium channels are open (which is effectively the same as not having sodium ions). Again we have a negative membrane potential. Similarly if only sodium channels are open, we have a positive membrane potential. Thus we can think of sodium and potassium channels are knobs for turning the membrane potential up and down. To keep the membrane voltage negative, as it is in the resting conditions, keep the potassium channels open, with sodium channels closed. To take the membrane potentials to positive levels, open the sodium channels and shut down the potassium channels. These intuitive considerations will be made more rigorous mathematically.

Ion Channels and Gating

We mentioned above that ion channels can be switched between OPEN and CLOSED states by various factors. This switching of the state of ion channels is known as gating.

There are 4 factors that drive channel gating: a) ligand-gating, b) voltage-gating, 3) phosphorylation c) stretch.

Ligand gating: In ligand-gating a molecule binds to the ion channel and changes its confirmation (shape), thereby changing its open/close state.

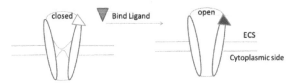

Ligand Gating

Voltage-gating: In this form of gating, it is the membrane voltage that controls channel gating. The fact that these channels are gated by voltage implies that their conductance is a function of membrane voltage. Therefore, the voltage-current characteristics of a voltage-gated or voltage-sensitive channel, are nonlinear. These channels do not obey the Ohm's law. These nonlinear conductances are crucial in generating neural signals in the form of sharp voltage spikes known as action potentials.

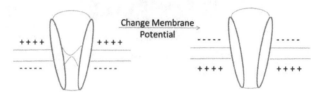

Voltage Gating

Phosphorylation-gating: In this form of gating, the channel goes to an open state form closed state when a phosphate group is attached to the channel, a process known as phosphorylation. The energy required for opening the channel comes from the phosphate group.

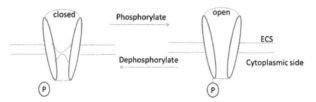

Phosphorylation Gating

Stretch-gating: Stretch of the cell membrane can also open channels. This mechanism converts a stretch event into an electrical event, since the opened channels permit current. Such channels are found, for example, in nerve endings that transduce touch in skin.

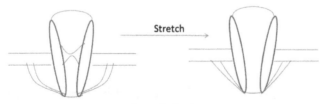

Stretch Gating

Each neuron receives signals via its dendrites, from other neurons; the dendritic signals flow towards the soma and combined at a part of the soma called the axon hillock; signals that arise from the axon hillock then propagate along the axon; at the end of the axon collaterals the axonal signals are transmitted to other neurons via the synapse. The cycle continues...

Thus, signaling in a neuron may be divided into four stages:

Stages of Neural Signaling

1) Signaling over the dendritic tree

2) Summation at the axon hillock

3) Signal propagation along the axon and its collaterals

4) Signal transmission across the synapse

Neural Signals are Electrical and Chemical:

So far we have been talking about neural "signals" rather vaguely without specifying the nature of these signals. Neural signals are electrical or chemical depending on the site of the signals. Among the 4 signaling components mentioned above, the first three are electrical, while the last one, signal transmission across the synapse, is a chemical step.

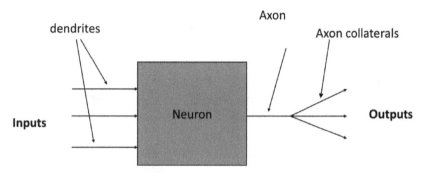

A neuron as an input/output system. Inputs from other neurons are received by the dendritic tree. Signals generated by a neuron are transmitted/broadcast to other neurons by the axon collaterals

Dendritic Signals

The signals that are received at a dendritic branch from the axon terminal of another neuron, via a synapse, is in the form of a local voltage change. This voltage change can be either positive or negative, depending on the nature of the synapse. This voltage deviation propagates, like a wave, towards the cell body. Propagation along a dendrite is lossy. Therefore, the wave as it propagates loses amplitude and widens in time. Different waves, positive and negative, originating at different times, at different locations on the dendritic tree, flow towards the soma and get summated there.

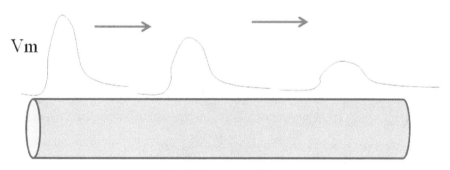

Dendritic propagation.

Summation at the Soma and Action Potential

The voltage waves arriving from the dendritic arbor, get summated at the soma, or more specifically the axon hillock, a knobby part of the soma at the root of the axon. The axon hillock has a high concentration of voltage-sensitive sodium and potassium channels, which is the reason behind a special response property of a neuron known as the "all-or-none" response. To illustrate this "all-or-none" response consider a thought-experiment in which you inject a pulse of current into a neuron. A small current pulse produces a small transient, upward deviation in the neuron voltage. As the current pulse amplitude is increased, amplitude of the voltage deviation also grows proportionally until the response reaches a threshold voltage level. Beyond this threshold, the neuron's voltage continues to increase rapidly up to a high value and sharply drops to the original resting potential. This transient, rapid rise and fall of neuron voltage is known as Action Potential (AP). It has 3 phases:

- Rising Phase

- Falling Phase

- After Hyperpolarisation

Refractory period of the AP is a short period of time after an action potential has occurred, the cell membrane cannot fire another action potential. This can be Absolute refractory period: voltage-gated Na+ channels won't open again or Relative refractory period: cell is hyperpolarized

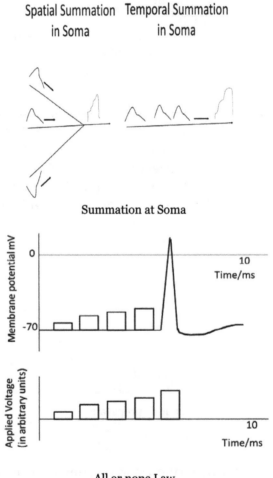

Spatial Summation in Soma   Temporal Summation in Soma

Summation at Soma

All or none Law

When voltage waves of different amplitudes and signs flow towards the soma, they add up to change the local voltage of the soma. If that change is positive and exceeds a threshold value, an AP is produced at the axon hillock. If the net voltage change does not exceed the threshold value, no AP is produced. The state in which a neuron produces an AP is known as an excited state, as opposed to the usual resting state of the neuron when the voltage is a low, constant value.

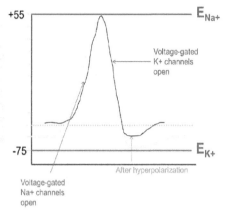

Phases in an Action Potential

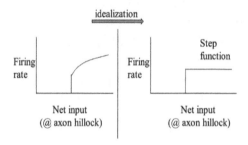

This simplification/idealization forms the basis for
construction of large network models

Neuron as a Thresholding Device

Axonal Propagation

The AP produced at the axon hillock propagates along the axon and reaches the axon collaterals. An important difference lies in the manner in which an AP propagates along the axon, and a voltage wave propagates along the dendrites. A voltage wave loses its amplitude and also spreads in time as it propagates down the dendritic tree towards the soma. But an AP propagates intact, without losing amplitude or spreading in time, as it propagates along an axon.

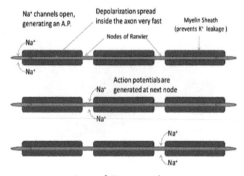

Axonal Propagation

This is possible because of presence of special molecular machinery on the axon and also in the axon hillock. This machinery is responsible for charging up the signal as it propagates along the cable.

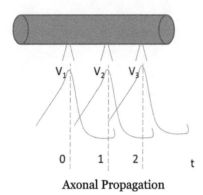

Axonal Propagation

Synapse

The synapse forms the functional connection between two neurons. It is a convenient window through which one neuron signals to another. The synapse is what makes the brain a network of neurons and not a mass of cells. Most importantly, it is the site of most learning and memory in the brain. It is now believed that whenever the brain learns something, the result of learning is somehow encoded in the properties of synapses. Recognition of the importance of the synapse in understanding brain function has led to a whole movement known as "Connectionism."

The synapse is a special structure where all the neurochemical machinery for neuron to neuron signaling is concentrated. Its design ensures that a signal released by a neuron has maximal effect on a target neuron with minimum attenuation. Based on the nature of signal used, synapses are classified as i) electrical synapses and ii) chemical synapses.

Electrical Synapses

Electrical synapses are direct cell-to-cell contacts. They are mediated by gap junctions, which form corridors that directly connect cytosols of two neurons. These corridors can permit passage of ions and small molecules. Thus two neurons coupled by gap junctions can electrically signal to each other by exchange of ions.

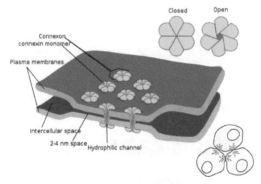

Electrical Synapse

Electrical synapses are typically bidirectional i.e., signal propagates in both directions(from neuron A to neuron B and back). This is because the electrical synapses may be simply regarded as a passive conductance that links the membrane voltages of two neurons. (There are, however, rectifying gap junctions in which conductance is greater in one direction than the other, analogous to a diode in electronic circuits. These may still be considered bidirectional with some asymmetry.)

Chemical Synapses

In a chemical synapse, signaling is mediated by a chemical messenger that transduces electrical changes in one neuron and translates it into appropriate electrical changes in a target neuron.

Some terminology is in line. Transmission across a chemical synapse is unidirectional proceeding from the presynaptic neuron to the postsynaptic neuron. Synapse is simply a site where the axon terminal of the presynaptic neuron, known as the presynaptic terminal, and an appropriate part of the postsynaptic neuron, known as the postsynaptic terminal, are held in close proximity. The pre- and post- synaptic terminals have no physical contact and are separated by a gap known as the synaptic cleft. The cleft is rather narrow with a gap of only about 20 nm. Such close apposition of the pre- and post-synaptic terminals in a synapse makes possible a reliable transmission with minimal loss.

Neurotransmission

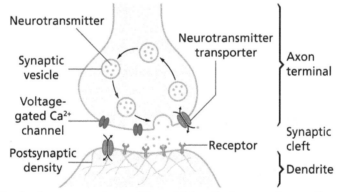

The presynaptic neuron (top) releases neurotransmitter, which activates receptors on the postsynaptic cell (bottom)

Neurotransmission (Latin: transmissio "passage, crossing" from transmittere "send, let through"), also called synaptic transmission, is the process by which signaling molecules called neurotransmitters are released by a neuron (the presynaptic neuron), and bind to and activate the receptors of another neuron (the postsynaptic neuron). Neurotransmission is essential for the process of communication between two neurons. Synaptic transmission relies on: the availability of the neurotransmitter; the release of the neurotransmitter by exocytosis; the binding of the postsynaptic receptor by the neurotransmitter; the functional response of the postsynaptic cell; and the subsequent removal or deactivation of the neurotransmitter.

In response to a threshold action potential or graded electrical potential, a neurotransmitter is released at the presynaptic terminal. The released neurotransmitter may then move across the synapse to be detected by and bind with receptors in the postsynaptic neuron. Binding of neurotransmitters may influence the postsynaptic neuron in either an inhibitory or excitatory way. The binding of neurotransmitters to receptors in the postsynaptic neuron can trigger either short term changes, such as changes in the membrane potential called postsynaptic potentials, or longer term changes by the activation of signaling cascades.

Neurons form elaborate networks through which nerve impulses (action potentials) travel. Each neuron has as many as 15,000 connections with other neurons. Neurons do not touch each other (except in the case of an electrical synapse through a gap junction); instead, neurons interact at close contact points called synapses. A neuron transports its information by way of an action potential. When the nerve impulse arrives at the synapse, it may cause the release of neurotransmitters, which influence another (postsynaptic) neuron. The postsynaptic neuron may receive inputs from many additional neurons, both excitatory and inhibitory. The excitatory and inhibitory influences are summed, and if the net effect is inhibitory, the neuron will be less likely to "fire" (i.e., generate an action potential), and if the net effect is excitatory, the neuron will be more likely to fire. How likely a neuron is to fire depends on how far its membrane potential is from the threshold potential, the voltage at which an action potential is triggered because enough voltage-dependent sodium channels are activated so that the net inward sodium current exceeds all outward currents. Excitatory inputs bring a neuron closer to threshold, while inhibitory inputs bring the neuron farther from threshold. An action potential is an "all-or-none" event; neurons whose membranes have not reached threshold will not fire, while those that do must fire. Once the action potential is initiated (traditionally at the axon hillock), it will propagate along the axon, leading to release of neurotransmitters at the synaptic bouton to pass along information to yet another adjacent neuron.

Stages in Neurotransmission at the Synapse

1. Synthesis of the neurotransmitter. This can take place in the cell body, in the axon, or in the axon terminal.

2. Storage of the neurotransmitter in storage granules or vesicles in the axon terminal.

3. Calcium enters the axon terminal during an action potential, causing release of the neurotransmitter into the synaptic cleft.

4. After its release, the transmitter binds to and activates a receptor in the postsynaptic membrane.

5. Deactivation of the neurotransmitter. The neurotransmitter is either destroyed enzymatically, or taken back into the terminal from which it came, where it can be reused, or degraded and removed.

General Description

Neurotransmitters are spontaneously packed in vesicles and released in individual quanta-packets independently of presynaptic action potentials. This slow release is detectable and produces micro-inhibitory or micro-excitatory effects on the postsynaptic neuron. An action potential briefly amplifies this process. Neurotransmitter containing vesicles cluster around active sites, and after they have been released may be recycled by one of three proposed mechanism. The first proposed mechanism involves partial opening and then re-closing of the vesicle. The second two involve the full fusion of the vesicle with the membrane, followed by recycling, or recycling into the endosome. Vesicular fusion is driven largely by the concentration of calcium in micro domains located near calcium channels, allowing for only microseconds of neurotransmitter release, while returning to normal calcium concentration takes a couple of hundred of microseconds. The vesicle exocytosis is through to be driven by a protein complex called SNARE, that is the target for botulinum toxins. Once released, a neurotransmitter enters the synapse and encounters receptors. Neurotransmitters receptors can either be inotropic or g protein coupled. Inotropic receptors allow for ions to pass through when agonized by a ligand. The main model involves a receptor composed of multiple subunits that allow for coordination of ion preference. G protein coupled receptors, also called metabotropic receptors, when bound to by a ligand undergo conformational changes yielding in intracellular response. Termination of neurotransmitter activity is usually done by a transporter, however enzymatic deactivation is also plausible.

Summation

Each neuron connects with numerous other neurons, receiving numerous impulses from them. Summation is the adding together of these impulses at the axon hillock. If the neuron only gets excitatory impulses, it will generate an action potential. If instead the neuron gets as many inhibitory as excitatory impulses, the inhibition cancels out the excitation and the nerve impulse will stop there. Action potential generation is proportionate to the probability and pattern of neurotransmitter release, and to postsynaptic receptor sensitization.

Spatial summation means that the effects of impulses received at different places on the neuron add up, so that the neuron may fire when such impulses are received simultaneously, even if each impulse on its own would not be sufficient to cause firing.

Temporal summation means that the effects of impulses received at the same place can add up if the impulses are received in close temporal succession. Thus the neuron may fire when multiple impulses are received, even if each impulse on its own would not be sufficient to cause firing.

Convergence and Divergence

Neurotransmission implies both a convergence and a divergence of information. First one neuron is influenced by many others, resulting in a convergence of input. When the neuron fires, the signal is sent to many other neurons, resulting in a divergence of output. Many other neurons are influenced by this neuron.

Cotransmission

Cotransmission is the release of several types of neurotransmitters from a single nerve terminal.

At the nerve terminal, neurotransmitters are present within 35–50 nm membrane-encased vesicles called synaptic vesicles. To release neurotransmitters, the synaptic vesicles transiently dock and fuse at the base of specialized 10–15 nm cup-shaped lipoprotein structures at the presynaptic membrane called porosomes. The neuronal porosome proteome has been solved, providing the molecular architecture and the complete composition of the machinery.

Recent studies in a myriad of systems have shown that most, if not all, neurons release several different chemical messengers. Cotransmission allows for more complex effects at postsynaptic receptors, and thus allows for more complex communication to occur between neurons.

In modern neuroscience, neurons are often classified by their cotransmitter. For example, striatal "GABAergic neurons" utilize opioid peptides or substance P as their primary cotransmitter.

Some neurons can release at least two neurotransmitters at the same time, the other being a cotransmitter, in order to provide the stabilizing negative feedback required for meaningful encoding, in the absence of inhibitory interneurons. Examples include:

- GABA–glycine co-release.

- Dopamine–glutamate co-release.

- Acetylcholine (Ach)–glutamate co-release.

- ACh–vasoactive intestinal peptide (VIP) co-release.

- ACh–calcitonin gene-related peptide (CGRP) co-release.

- Glutamate–dynorphin co-release (in hippocampus).

Genetic Association

Neurotransmission is genetically associated with other characteristics or features. For example, enrichment analyses of different signaling pathways led to the discovery of a genetic association with intracranial volume.

As mentioned above signaling processes up to the time when an AP arrives at an axon terminal are electrical, while the signal transmission across the synapse involves exchange of chemicals. When an AP arrives at an axon terminal, a special substance, known as the neurotransmitter, is released from the terminal, by exocytosis. This release is probabilistic and every AP need not produce a PSP. The neurotransmitter diffuses through a 20 nm gap contained in the synapse, known as the synaptic cleft, and reaches the dendrite of another neuron.

Action of neurotransmitter on the dendrite produces a voltage change in the dendrite known as the Post Synaptic Potential. This is simply the positive or negative deviation from the membrane potential of the dendrite, as described above. A positive voltage is more likely to propagate to soma and increase its local voltage, contributing its subsequent excitation. Therefore, a positive change is known as the Excitatory Post Synaptic Potential (EPSP). On the other hand, a negative change, when it propagates to the soma, tends to prevent the neuron from excitation. In other words, it tends to inhibit the neuron. Therefore, such voltage change is known as the Inhibitory Post Synaptic Potential (IPSP). A synapse at which a EPSP is produced is called an excitatory synapse while the synapse at which an IPSP is produced is an inhibitory synapse. Now let us take a closer look at the process of neurotransmission. What makes one transmission event produce an EPSP as opposed to an IPSP? There are three molecular players in the process of neurotransmission: neurotransmitter, receptor and an ion channel. When the transmitter molecules released from the presynaptic terminal diffuse towards the postsynaptic terminal and bind with a receptor, which is associated with an ion channel. The binding event between the neurotransmitter and the receptor opens the associated ion channel. If the channel that is opened is a Na⁺ channel, the local, postsynaptic membrane potential increases, which is the EPSP. On the other hand, when the ion channel that is opened is a K⁺ or a Cl⁻ channel, it results in a negative deviation in the postsynaptic membrane voltage, which is an IPSP.

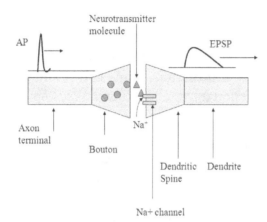

Excitatorry Post Synaptic Potential (EPSP)

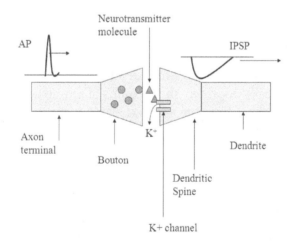

Inhibitory Post Synaptic Potential (IPSP)

Let us consider a few basic facts about neurotransmitter, receptor and ion channels.

Neurotransmitter

In terms of their action, neurotransmitters may be broadly classified into excitatory and inhibitory neurotransmitters. A neurotransmitter that produces an EPSP is known as an excitatory neurotransmitter, an important example of which is glutamate. Similarly a neurotransmitter that produces an IPSP is an inhibitory neurotransmitter, a key example of which is Gamma Aminobutyric Acid (GABA). Glutamate and GABA are two important neurotransmitters in the brain. Over half of all brain synapses release glutamate, and about 30-40% of all brain synapses release GABA. Increased glutamate transmission tends to increase the overall excitation in the brain, while GABA transmission has the opposite effect. The push-pull effect due to glutamate and GABA keep the brain in a state of balance between over-excitation and total inhibition.

Neurotransmitters vary in terms of their speed of action, scope of action, spatial extent of their action etc. However, in terms of chemistry, the classes of neurotransmitters: i) amino acids, ii) biogenic amines, iii) others and iv) neuropeptides.

The below three categories of neurotransmitter are grouped under the general class of fast-acting neurotransmitters, since their post-synaptic effects show up at the time scales of milliseconds.

   i)   Amino Acids: There are 4 main candidates in this category: glutamate, aspartate, amino-butyric acid (GABA) and glycine. These are fast acting, capable of producing post-synaptic currents within a few milliseconds. Glutamate and aspartate are prominent excitatory transmitters, while GABA and glycine are inhibitory. Most rapid neurotransmission in vertebrate nervous systems is mediated by this class of neurotransmitters.

   ii)   Biogenic Amines: There are 5 substances in this category: acetylcholine (Ach), norepinephrine, dopamine, serotonin and histamine. Their activity is much slower than the amino acid neurotransmitters, lasting over a duration of hundreds of milliseconds. However, as it is almost always the case in biology, there are exceptions. The speed of transmission depends on the type of receptor. For example, Acetylcholine acts fast when the transmission in mediate by a nicotinic receptor and slow acting in case of a muscaranic receptor.

   iii)   Others: adenosine, nitric oxide etc.

In addition to the above 3 classes, there is another broad class of neurotransmitters known as neuropeptides. These are basically peptides, short chains of amino acids, which can have action on the postsynaptic side. The neuropeptides are said to be slow-acting since their postsynaptic action occurs over time scales of seconds.

   iv)   Neuropeptides β-endorphin is an important example of a neuropeptide which interacts with opioid receptors in the brain. These are short chains of amino acids, acting over a time scale of minutes or more. This class of neurotransmitters is sometimes present along with ("colocalized") with other fast-acting neutransmitters. Release of this type of neurotransmitter occurs at a greater firing rate of the presynaptic stimulus, compared to what it takes to release fast acting neurotransmitters.

A question that often arises regarding neurotransmitters is: does a synapse release a single neurotransmitter or multiple neurotransmitters? A general principle of neurotransmission, called Dale's principle, states that a neuron releases only a single transmitter. This is not true since a single neuron can release multiple transmitters from its synapses, a phenomenon known as cotransmission. Thus a modified form of Dale's principle, due to Sir John Eccles, states that "at all the axonal branches of a neuron, there was liberation of the same transmitter substance or substances." Thus the same set of neurotransmitters are released by a neuron throughout its lifetime at its synapses.

Receptors

Receptors are grouped as 1) ionotropic or 2) metabotrophic receptors, based on the manner in which they interact with the associated ion channel.

1) In ionotropic receptors, the receptor or the binding site is located on another part of the protein complex that forms the ion channel.

2) In metabotrophic receptors, the biding of neurotransmitter and receptor activates a series of intra-cellular events, one of which is the channel opening.

A given neurotransmitter can have several receptors.

Examples:

1) Glutamate receptors: 3 ionotropic and 1 metabotropic.

    a. Ionotropic receptors: N-methyl D-aspartate (NMDA) receptor, α-amino-3- hydroxyl-5-methyl-4-isoxazole-propionate (AMPA) receptor, kainate receptor.

    b. Metabotropic receptor: mGluR receptor.

2) GABA receptors: are of two classes.

    a. GABAa receptors are ionotropic

    b. GABAb receptors are metabotropic

Structural Classification of Synapses

Above we described a synapse structurally as a meeting point between axon terminal of the presynaptic neuron and an "appropriate part" of the post-synaptic neuron. Synapses are actually classified on the basis of what this "appropriate part" of the post-synaptic neuron is:

    1) Axodendritic synapses: These synapses occur between axon terminals of one neuron and a dendrite of another. Further, this contact can occur at the shaft of the dendrite, or at a dendritic spine. It has been observed that synapses on dendritic spines are usually excitatory. When a signal is transmitted across an axodendritic synapse it undergoes certain attenuation as it propagates down the dendritic tree towards the soma of the post- synaptic neuron. This propagation also involves a certain delay.

    2) Axosomatic synapses: In these synapses, the axon terminal of one neuron makes contact with the soma of another. Typically these synapses happen to be inhibitory. By virtue of their proximity to the soma, signals across axosomatic synapses are more effective than signals from axodendritic synapses.

    3) Axoaxonic synapses: Existence of axoaxonic synapses seems counterintuitive since a synapse is supposed to be junction between the output end of a neuron (its axon terminal) and the input end (dendrite or soma) of another neuron. However such synapses do exist. Signal across an axoaxonic synapse typically modulates transmission across one of the above two types of neurons.

Synaptic Transmission

To summarize, a synapse simply converts an electrical event on the pre- side (arrival of AP) into an electrical event on the post- side (EPSP or IPSP). This conversion is done by an intermediate chemical step mediated by the trinity of Neurotransmitter-Receptor-Ion Channel. Figure shows the major structural components of a chemical synapse.

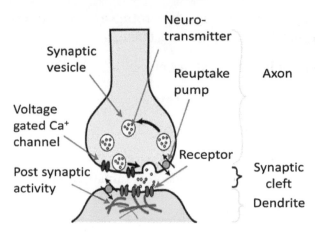

Major structural components of a synapse

How does this transformation of an AP on the pre- side to a PSP on the post- side take place? Complex molecular machinery is used for this purpose. Let us a take a closer look at the series of events involved in this conversion.

Step 1: AP generated at the axon hillock arrives at the axon terminal or the pre-synaptic terminal.

Step 2: AP arrival increases local membrane potential in the pre-synaptic terminal.

Step 3: Voltage-sensitive Ca^{++} channels open. Ca^{++} rushes into the pre-synaptic terminal.

Step 4: Increased Ca^{++} concentration in the pre-synaptic terminal causes vesicles containing neurotransmitter to fuse with pre-synaptic membrane and release neurotransmitter into the synaptic cleft. Such spewing out of material by cells is known as exocytosis.

Step 5: Neurotransmitter diffuses through the synaptic cleft and binds to receptor molecules on the post-synaptic membrane.

Step 6: The binding event signals to associated ion channels to open/close.

Step 7: Current influx/efflux through the open channels produces a (E/I)PSP across the post-synaptic membrane.

There are certain secondary, "clean up" events that accompany the above events.

Step 4b: (Vesicle recycling): When vesicles fuse with the pre-synaptic membrane, the membrane of the vesicle fuses with plasma membrane increasing the surface area of the pre-synaptic membrane. If this process goes on indefinitely, there will not be any membrane left for synthesis of new vesicles. However, the vesicular membrane patch that fused with the pre-synaptic membrane is recycled, taken back into the pre-synaptic terminal for synthesizing new vesicles. This process is thought to occur via several intricate mechanisms.

Step 5b: Transmitter molecules that are released into the synaptic cleft do not linger there for ever. They are removed from that region by several mechanisms. This removal is necessary to terminate the transmission process. Otherwise prolonged exposure of post- synaptic receptors to transmitter molecules makes the receptors insensitive to subsequent signals coming from the pre-synaptic side. Removal of transmitter from the cleft is done by 3 mechanisms: 1) diffusion, 2) enzymatic degradation (breaking down of transmitter by specific enzymes) and 3) re-uptake (transmitter molecules are actively taken back into pre-synaptic terminals and packaged into newly synthesized vesicles).

Synaptic Strength

Since the PSP produced as a result of a single AP on the presynaptic side has variable magnitude, we can introduce the notion of synaptic strength. There is no single, textbook definition of synaptic strength. Biologically speaking there are several factors, both pre- and post-synaptic, that determine the synaptic strength. A reasonable definition of synaptic strength could be:

Synaptic strength = average PSP produced in response to an AP on the presynaptic side.

Synaptic strength figures as an important quantity in any discussion of information processing in the brain, since this strength varies as an effect of learning and memory. Results of learning and memory seem to be coded in the form of synaptic strength. This labile quality of synapses is known as synaptic plasticity.

Nervous System

The nervous system is the part of an animal's body that coordinates its actions and transmits signals to and from different parts of its body. Nervous tissue first arose in wormlike organisms about 550 to 600 million years ago. In vertebrate species it consists of two main parts, the central nervous system (CNS) and the peripheral nervous system (PNS). The CNS contains the brain and spinal cord. The PNS consists mainly of nerves, which are enclosed bundles of the long fibers or axons, that connect the CNS to every other part of the body. Nerves that transmit signals from the brain are called motor or efferent nerves, while those nerves that transmit information from the body to the CNS are called sensory or afferent. Most nerves serve both functions and are called mixed nerves. The PNS is divided into a) somatic and b) autonomic nervous system, and c) the enteric nervous system. Somatic nerves mediate voluntary movement. The autonomic nervous system is further subdivided into the sympathetic and the parasympathetic nervous systems. The sympathetic nervous system is activated in cases of emergencies to mobilize energy, while the parasympathetic nervous system is activated when organisms are in a relaxed state. The enteric nervous system functions to control the gastrointestinal system. Both autonomic and enteric nervous systems function involuntarily. Nerves that exit from the cranium are called cranial nerves while those exiting from the spinal cord are called spinal nerves.

At the cellular level, the nervous system is defined by the presence of a special type of cell, called the neuron, also known as a "nerve cell". Neurons have special structures that allow them to send signals rapidly and precisely to other cells. They send these signals in the form of electrochemical waves traveling along thin fibers called axons, which cause chemicals called neurotransmitters to be released at junctions called synapses. A cell that receives a synaptic signal from a neuron may be excited, inhibited, or otherwise modulated. The connections between neurons can form neural circuits and also neural networks that generate an organism's perception of the world and determine its behavior. Along with neurons, the nervous system contains other specialized cells called glial cells (or simply glia), which provide structural and metabolic support.

Nervous systems are found in most multicellular animals, but vary greatly in complexity. The only multicellular animals that have no nervous system at all are sponges, placozoans, and mesozoans, which have very simple body plans. The nervous systems of the radially symmetric organisms ctenophores (comb jellies) and cnidarians (which include anemones, hydras, corals and jellyfish) consist of a diffuse nerve net. All other animal species, with the exception of a few types of worm, have a nervous system containing a brain, a central cord (or two cords running in parallel), and nerves radiating from the brain and central cord. The size of the nervous system ranges from a few hundred cells in the simplest worms, to around 300 billion cells in African elephants.

The central nervous system functions to send signals from one cell to others, or from one part of the body to others and to receive feedback. Malfunction of the nervous system can occur as a result of genetic defects, physical damage due to trauma or toxicity, infection or simply of ageing. The medical specialty of neurology studies disorders of the nervous system and looks for interventions that can prevent or treat them. In the peripheral nervous system, the most common problem is the failure of nerve conduction, which can be due to different causes including diabetic neuropathy and demyelinating disorders such as multiple sclerosis and amyotrophic lateral sclerosis. Neuroscience is the field of science that focuses on the study of the nervous system.

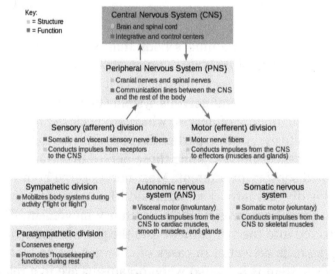

Diagram showing the major divisions of the vertebrate nervous system

Structure

The nervous system derives its name from nerves, which are cylindrical bundles of fibers (the axons of neurons), that emanate from the brain and spinal cord, and branch repeatedly to innervate every part of the body. Nerves are large enough to have been recognized by the ancient Egyptians, Greeks, and Romans, but their internal structure was not understood until it became possible to examine them using a microscope. "It is difficult to believe that until approximately year 1900 it was not known that neurons are the basic units of the brain (Santiago Ramón y Cajal). Equally surprising is the fact that the concept of chemical transmission in the brain was not known until around 1930 (Henry Hallett Dale) and (Otto Loewi). We began to understand the basic electrical phenomenon that neurons use in order to communicate among themselves, the action potential, in the 1950s (Alan Lloyd Hodgkin, Andrew Huxley and John Eccles). It was in the 1960s that we became aware of how basic neuronal networks code stimuli and thus basic concepts are possible (David H. Hubel, and Torsten Wiesel). The molecular revolution swept across US universities in the 1980s. It was in the 1990s that molecular mechanisms of behavioral phenomena became widely known (Eric Richard Kandel)." A microscopic examination shows that nerves consist primarily of axons, along with different membranes that wrap around them and segregate them into fascicles. The neurons that give rise to nerves do not lie entirely within the nerves themselves—their cell bodies reside within the brain, spinal cord, or peripheral ganglia.

All animals more advanced than sponges have nervous systems. However, even sponges, unicellular animals, and non-animals such as slime molds have cell-to-cell signalling mechanisms that are precursors to those of neurons. In radially symmetric animals such as the jellyfish and hydra, the nervous system consists of a nerve net, a diffuse network of isolated cells. In bilaterian animals, which make up the great majority of existing species, the nervous system has a common structure that originated early in the Ediacaran period, over 550 million years ago.

Cells

The nervous system contains two main categories or types of cells: neurons and glial cells.

Neurons

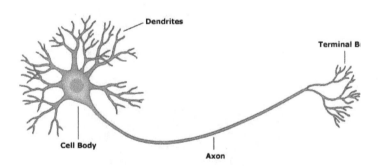

The nervous system is defined by the presence of a special type of cell—the neuron (sometimes called "neurone" or "nerve cell"). Neurons can be distinguished from other cells in a number of ways, but their most fundamental property is that they communicate with other cells via synapses, which are membrane-to-membrane junctions containing molecular machinery that allows rapid transmission of signals, either electrical or chemical. Many types of neuron possess an axon, a protoplasmic protrusion that can extend to distant parts of the body and make thousands of synaptic contacts. Axons frequently travel through the body in bundles called nerves.

Even in the nervous system of a single species such as humans, hundreds of different types of neurons exist, with a wide variety of morphologies and functions. These include sensory neurons that transmute physical stimuli such as light and sound into neural signals, and motor neurons that transmute neural signals into activation of muscles or glands; however in many species the great majority of neurons participate in the formation of centralized structures (the brain and ganglia) and they receive all of their input from other neurons and send their output to other neurons.

Glial Cells

Glial cells are non-neuronal cells that provide support and nutrition, maintain homeostasis, form myelin, and participate in signal transmission in the nervous system. In the human brain, it is estimated that the total number of glia roughly equals the number of neurons, although the proportions vary in different brain areas. Among the most important functions of glial cells are to support neurons and hold them in place; to supply nutrients to neurons; to insulate neurons electrically; to destroy pathogens and remove dead neurons; and to provide guidance cues directing the axons of neurons to their targets. A very important type of glial cell (oligodendrocytes in the central nervous system, and Schwann cells in the peripheral nervous system) generates layers of a fatty substance called myelin that wraps around axons and provides electrical insulation which allows them to transmit action potentials much more rapidly and efficiently. Recent findings indicate that glial cells, such as microglia and astrocytes, serve as important resident immune cells within the central nervous system.

Anatomy in Vertebrates

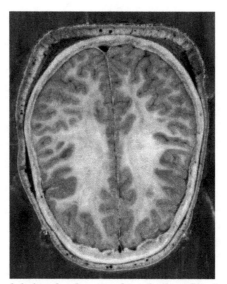

Horizontal section of the head of an adult female, showing skin, skull, and brain with grey matter (brown in this image) and underlying white matter

The nervous system of vertebrates (including humans) is divided into the central nervous system (CNS) and the peripheral nervous system (PNS).

The (CNS) is the major division, and consists of the brain and the spinal cord. The spinal canal contains the spinal cord, while the cranial cavity contains the brain. The CNS is enclosed and protected by the meninges, a three-layered system of membranes, including a tough, leathery outer layer called the dura mater. The brain is also protected by the skull, and the spinal cord by the vertebrae.

The peripheral nervous system (PNS) is a collective term for the nervous system structures that do not lie within the CNS. The large majority of the axon bundles called nerves are considered to belong to the PNS, even when the cell bodies of the neurons to which they belong reside within the brain or spinal cord. The PNS is divided into somatic and visceral parts. The somatic part consists of the nerves that innervate the skin, joints, and muscles. The cell bodies of somatic sensory neurons lie in dorsal root ganglia of the spinal cord. The visceral part, also known as the autonomic nervous system, contains neurons that innervate the internal organs, blood vessels, and glands. The autonomic nervous system itself consists of two parts: the sympathetic nervous system and the parasympathetic nervous system. Some authors also include sensory neurons whose cell bodies lie in the periphery (for senses such as hearing) as part of the PNS; others, however, omit them.

The vertebrate nervous system can also be divided into areas called grey matter ("gray matter" in American spelling) and white matter. Grey matter (which is only grey in preserved tissue, and is better described as pink or light brown in living tissue) contains a high proportion of cell bodies of neurons. White matter is composed mainly of myelinated axons, and takes its color from the myelin. White matter includes all of the nerves, and much of the interior of the brain and spinal cord. Grey matter is found in clusters of neurons in the brain and spinal cord, and in cortical layers that line their surfaces. There is an anatomical convention that a cluster of neurons in the brain or spinal cord is called a nucleus, whereas a cluster of neurons in the periphery is called a ganglion. There are, however, a few exceptions to this rule, notably including the part of the forebrain called the basal ganglia.

Comparative Anatomy and Evolution

Neural Precursors in Sponges

Sponges have no cells connected to each other by synaptic junctions, that is, no neurons, and therefore no nervous system. They do, however, have homologs of many genes that play key roles in synaptic function. Recent studies have shown that sponge cells express a group of proteins that cluster together to form a structure resembling a postsynaptic density (the signal-receiving part of a synapse). However, the function of this structure is currently unclear. Although sponge cells do not show synaptic transmission, they do communicate with each other via calcium waves and other impulses, which mediate some simple actions such as whole-body contraction.

Radiata

Jellyfish, comb jellies, and related animals have diffuse nerve nets rather than a central nervous system. In most jellyfish the nerve net is spread more or less evenly across the body; in comb jellies it is concentrated near the mouth. The nerve nets consist of sensory neurons, which pick up chemical, tactile, and visual signals; motor neurons, which can activate contractions of the body wall; and intermediate neurons, which detect patterns of activity in the sensory neurons and, in response, send signals to groups of motor neurons. In some cases groups of intermediate neurons are clustered into discrete ganglia.

The development of the nervous system in radiata is relatively unstructured. Unlike bilaterians, radiata only have two primordial cell layers, endoderm and ectoderm. Neurons are generated from a special set of ectodermal precursor cells, which also serve as precursors for every other ectodermal cell type.

Bilateria

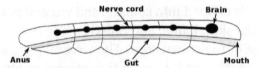

Nervous system of a bilaterian animal, in the form of a nerve cord with segmental enlargements, and a "brain" at the front

The vast majority of existing animals are bilaterians, meaning animals with left and right sides that are approximate mirror images of each other. All bilateria are thought to have descended from a common wormlike ancestor that appeared in the Ediacaran period, 550–600 million years ago. The fundamental bilaterian body form is a tube with a hollow gut cavity running from mouth to anus, and a nerve cord with an enlargement (a "ganglion") for each body segment, with an especially large ganglion at the front, called the "brain".

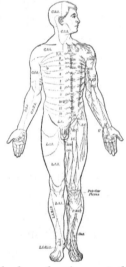

Area of the human body surface innervated by each spinal nerve

Even mammals, including humans, show the segmented bilaterian body plan at the level of the nervous system. The spinal cord contains a series of segmental ganglia, each giving rise to motor and sensory nerves that innervate a portion of the body surface and underlying musculature. On the limbs, the layout of the innervation pattern is complex, but on the trunk it gives rise to a series of narrow bands. The top three segments belong to the brain, giving rise to the forebrain, midbrain, and hindbrain.

Bilaterians can be divided, based on events that occur very early in embryonic development, into two groups (superphyla) called protostomes and deuterostomes. Deuterostomes include vertebrates as well as echinoderms, hemichordates (mainly acorn worms), and Xenoturbellidans. Protostomes, the more diverse group, include arthropods, molluscs, and numerous types of worms. There is a basic difference between the two groups in the placement of the nervous system within the body: protostomes possess a nerve cord on the ventral (usually bottom) side of the body, whereas in deuterostomes the nerve cord is on the dorsal (usually top) side. In fact, numerous aspects of the body are inverted between the two groups, including the expression patterns of several genes that show dorsal-to-ventral gradients. Most anatomists now consider that the bodies of protostomes and deuterostomes are "flipped over" with respect to each other, a hypothesis that was first proposed by Geoffroy Saint-Hilaire for insects in comparison to vertebrates. Thus insects, for example, have nerve cords that run along the ventral midline of the body, while all vertebrates have spinal cords that run along the dorsal midline.

Worms

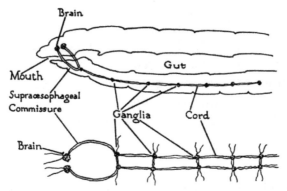

Earthworm nervous system. *Top:* side view of the front of the worm. *Bottom:* nervous system in isolation, viewed from above

Worms are the simplest bilaterian animals, and reveal the basic structure of the bilaterian nervous system in the most straightforward way. As an example, earthworms have dual nerve cords running along the length of the body and merging at the tail and the mouth. These nerve cords are connected by transverse nerves like the rungs of a ladder. These transverse nerves help coordinate the two sides of the animal. Two ganglia at the head (the "nerve ring") end function similar to a simple brain. Photoreceptors on the animal's eyespots provide sensory information on light and dark.

The nervous system of one very small roundworm, the nematode *Caenorhabditis elegans*, has been completely mapped out in a connectome including its synapses. Every neuron and its cellular lineage has been recorded and most, if not all, of the neural connections are known. In this species, the nervous system is sexually dimorphic; the nervous systems of the two sexes, males and female hermaphrodites, have different numbers of neurons and groups of neurons that perform sex-specific functions. In *C. elegans*, males have exactly 383 neurons, while hermaphrodites have exactly 302 neurons.

Arthropods

Arthropods, such as insects and crustaceans, have a nervous system made up of a series of ganglia, connected by a ventral nerve cord made up of two parallel connectives running along the length of the belly. Typically, each body segment has one ganglion on each side, though some ganglia are fused to form the brain and other large ganglia. The head segment contains the brain, also known as the supraesophageal ganglion. In the insect nervous system, the brain is anatomically divided into the protocerebrum, deutocerebrum, and tritocerebrum. Immediately behind the brain is the subesophageal ganglion, which is composed of three pairs of fused ganglia. It controls the mouthparts, the salivary glands and certain muscles. Many arthropods have well-developed sensory organs, including compound eyes for vision and antennae for olfaction and pheromone sensation. The sensory information from these organs is processed by the brain.

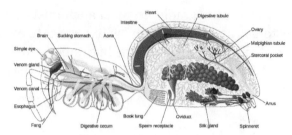

Internal anatomy of a spider, showing the nervous system in blue

In insects, many neurons have cell bodies that are positioned at the edge of the brain and are electrically passive—the cell bodies serve only to provide metabolic support and do not participate in signalling. A protoplasmic fiber runs from the cell body and branches profusely, with some parts transmitting signals and other parts receiving signals. Thus, most parts of the insect brain have passive cell bodies arranged around the periphery, while the neural signal processing takes place in a tangle of protoplasmic fibers called neuropil, in the interior.

"Identified" Neurons

A neuron is called *identified* if it has properties that distinguish it from every other neuron in the same animal—properties such as location, neurotransmitter, gene expression pattern, and connectivity—and if every individual organism belonging to the same species has one and only one neuron with the same set of properties. In vertebrate nervous systems very few neurons are "identified" in this sense—in humans, there are believed to be none—but in simpler nervous systems, some or all neurons may be thus unique. In the roundworm *C. elegans*, whose nervous system is the most thoroughly described of any animal's, every neuron in the body is uniquely identifiable, with the same location and the same connections in every individual worm. One notable consequence of this fact is that the form of the *C. elegans* nervous system is completely specified by the genome, with no experience-dependent plasticity.

The brains of many molluscs and insects also contain substantial numbers of identified neurons. In vertebrates, the best known identified neurons are the gigantic Mauthner cells of fish. Every fish has two Mauthner cells, located in the bottom part of the brainstem, one on the left side and one on the right. Each Mauthner cell has an axon that crosses over, innervating neurons at the same brain level and then travelling down through the spinal cord, making numerous connections as it goes. The synapses generated by a Mauthner cell are so powerful that a single action potential gives rise to a major behavioral response: within milliseconds the fish curves its body into a C-shape, then straightens, thereby propelling itself rapidly forward. Functionally this is a fast escape response, triggered most easily by a strong sound wave or pressure wave impinging on the lateral line organ of the fish. Mauthner cells are not the only identified neurons in fish—there are about 20 more types, including pairs of "Mauthner cell analogs" in each spinal segmental nucleus. Although a Mauthner cell is capable of bringing about an escape response individually, in the context of ordinary behavior other types of cells usually contribute to shaping the amplitude and direction of the response.

Mauthner cells have been described as command neurons. A command neuron is a special type of identified neuron, defined as a neuron that is capable of driving a specific behavior individually. Such neurons appear most commonly in the fast escape systems of various species—the squid giant axon and squid giant synapse, used for pioneering experiments in neurophysiology because of their enormous size, both participate in the fast escape circuit of the squid. The concept of a command neuron has, however, become controversial, because of studies showing that some neurons that initially appeared to fit the description were really only capable of evoking a response in a limited set of circumstances.

Function

At the most basic level, the function of the nervous system is to send signals from one cell to others, or from one part of the body to others. There are multiple ways that a cell can send signals to other cells. One is by releasing chemicals called hormones into the internal circulation, so that they can diffuse to distant sites. In contrast to this "broadcast" mode of signaling, the nervous system provides "point-to-point" signals—neurons project their axons to specific target areas and make synaptic connections with specific target cells. Thus, neural signaling is capable of a much higher level of specificity than hormonal signaling. It is also much faster: the fastest nerve signals travel at speeds that exceed 100 meters per second.

At a more integrative level, the primary function of the nervous system is to control the body. It does this by extracting information from the environment using sensory receptors, sending signals that encode this information into the central nervous system, processing the information to determine an appropriate response, and sending output signals to muscles or glands to activate the response. The evolution of a complex nervous system has made it possible for various animal species to have advanced perception abilities such as vision, complex social interactions, rapid coordination of organ systems, and integrated processing of concurrent signals. In humans, the sophistication of the nervous system makes it possible to have language, abstract representation of concepts, transmission of culture, and many other features of human society that would not exist without the human brain.

Neurons and Synapses

Most neurons send signals via their axons, although some types are capable of dendrite-to-dendrite communication. (In fact, the types of neurons called amacrine cells have no axons, and communicate only via their dendrites.) Neural signals propagate along an axon in the form of electrochemical waves called action potentials, which produce cell-to-cell signals at points where axon terminals make synaptic contact with other cells.

Synapses may be electrical or chemical. Electrical synapses make direct electrical connections between neurons, but chemical synapses are much more common, and much more diverse in function. At a chemical synapse, the cell that sends signals is called presynaptic, and the cell that receives signals is called postsynaptic. Both the presynaptic and postsynaptic areas are full of molecular machinery that carries out the signalling process. The presynaptic area contains large numbers of tiny spherical vessels called synaptic vesicles, packed with neurotransmitter chemicals. When the presynaptic terminal is electrically stimulated, an array of molecules embedded in the membrane are activated, and cause the contents of the vesicles to be released into the narrow space between the presynaptic and postsynaptic membranes, called the synaptic cleft. The neurotransmitter then binds to receptors embedded in the postsynaptic membrane, causing them to enter an activated state. Depending on the type of receptor, the resulting effect on the postsynaptic cell may be excitatory, inhibitory, or modulatory in more complex ways. For example, release of the neurotransmitter acetylcholine at a synaptic contact between a motor neuron and a muscle cell induces rapid contraction of the muscle cell. The entire synaptic transmission process takes only a fraction of a millisecond, although the effects on the postsynaptic cell may last much longer (even indefinitely, in cases where the synaptic signal leads to the formation of a memory trace).

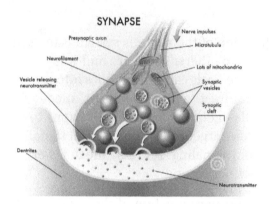

There are literally hundreds of different types of synapses. In fact, there are over a hundred known neurotransmitters, and many of them have multiple types of receptors. Many synapses use more than one neurotransmitter—a common arrangement is for a synapse to use one fast-acting small-molecule neurotransmitter such as glutamate or GABA, along with one or more peptide neurotransmitters that play slower-acting modulatory roles. Molecular neuroscientists generally divide receptors into two broad groups: chemically gated ion channels and second messenger systems. When a chemically gated ion channel is activated, it forms a passage that allows specific types of ions to flow across the membrane. Depending on the type of ion, the effect on the target cell may be excitatory or inhibitory. When a second messenger system is activated, it starts a cascade of molecular interactions inside the target cell, which may ultimately produce a wide variety of complex effects, such as increasing or decreasing the sensitivity of the cell to stimuli, or even altering gene transcription.

According to a rule called Dale's principle, which has only a few known exceptions, a neuron releases the same neurotransmitters at all of its synapses. This does not mean, though, that a neuron exerts the same effect on all of its targets, because the effect of a synapse depends not on the neurotransmitter, but on the receptors that it activates. Because different targets can (and frequently do) use different types of receptors, it is possible for a neuron to have excitatory effects on one set of target cells, inhibitory effects on others, and complex modulatory effects on others still. Nevertheless, it happens that the two most widely used neurotransmitters, glutamate and GABA, each have largely consistent effects. Glutamate has several widely occurring types of receptors, but all of them are excitatory or modulatory. Similarly, GABA has several widely occurring receptor types, but all of them are inhibitory. Because of this consistency, glutamatergic cells are frequently referred to as "excitatory neurons", and GABAergic cells as "inhibitory neurons". Strictly speaking, this is an abuse of terminology—it is the receptors that are excitatory and inhibitory, not the neurons—but it is commonly seen even in scholarly.

One very important subset of synapses are capable of forming memory traces by means of long-lasting activity-dependent changes in synaptic strength. The best-known form of neural memory is a process called long-term potentiation (abbreviated LTP), which operates at synapses that use the neurotransmitter glutamate acting on a special type of receptor known as the NMDA receptor. The NMDA receptor has an "associative" property: if the two cells involved in the synapse are both activated at approximately the same time, a channel opens that permits calcium to flow into the target cell. The calcium entry initiates a second messenger cascade that ultimately leads to an increase in the number of glutamate receptors in the target cell, thereby increasing the effective strength of the synapse. This change in strength can last for weeks or longer. Since the discovery of LTP in 1973, many other types of synaptic memory traces have been found, involving increases or decreases in synaptic strength that are induced by varying conditions, and last for variable periods of time. The reward system, that reinforces desired behaviour for example, depends on a variant form of LTP that is conditioned on an extra input coming from a reward-signalling pathway that uses dopamine as neurotransmitter. All these forms of synaptic modifiability, taken collectively, give rise to neural plasticity, that is, to a capability for the nervous system to adapt itself to variations in the environment.

Neural Circuits and Systems

The basic neuronal function of sending signals to other cells includes a capability for neurons to exchange signals with each other. Networks formed by interconnected groups of neurons are capable of a wide variety of functions, including feature detection, pattern generation and timing, and there are seen to be countless types of information processing possible. Warren McCulloch and Walter Pitts showed in 1943 that even artificial neural networks formed from a greatly simplified mathematical abstraction of a neuron are capable of universal computation.

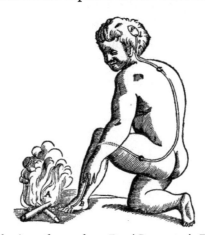

Illustration of pain pathway, from René Descartes's *Treatise of Man*

Historically, for many years the predominant view of the function of the nervous system was as a stimulus-response associator. In this conception, neural processing begins with stimuli that activate sensory neurons, producing signals that propagate through chains of connections in the spinal cord and brain, giving rise eventually to activation of motor neurons and thereby to muscle contraction, i.e., to overt responses. Descartes believed that all of the behaviors of animals, and most of the behaviors of humans, could be explained in terms of stimulus-response circuits, although he also believed that higher cognitive functions such as language were not capable of being explained mechanistically. Charles Sherrington, in his influential 1906 book *The Integrative Action of the Nervous System*, developed the concept of stimulus-response mechanisms in much more detail, and Behaviorism, the school of thought that dominated Psychology through the middle of the 20th century, attempted to explain every aspect of human behavior in stimulus-response terms.

However, experimental studies of electrophysiology, beginning in the early 20th century and reaching high productivity by the 1940s, showed that the nervous system contains many mechanisms for generating patterns of activity intrinsically, without requiring an external stimulus. Neurons were found to be capable of producing regular sequences of action potentials, or sequences of bursts, even in complete isolation. When intrinsically active neurons are connected to each other in complex circuits, the possibilities for generating intricate temporal patterns become far more extensive. A modern conception views the function of the nervous system partly in terms of stimulus-response chains, and partly in terms of intrinsically generated activity patterns—both types of activity interact with each other to generate the full repertoire of behavior.

Reflexes and Other Stimulus-response Circuits

The simplest type of neural circuit is a reflex arc, which begins with a sensory input and ends with a motor output, passing through a sequence of neurons connected in series. This can be shown in the "withdrawal reflex" causing a hand to jerk back after a hot stove is touched. The circuit begins with sensory receptors in the skin that are activated by harmful levels of heat: a special type of molecular structure embedded in the membrane causes heat to change the electrical field across the membrane. If the change in electrical potential is large enough to pass the given threshold, it evokes an action potential, which is transmitted along the axon of the receptor cell, into the spinal cord. There the axon makes excitatory synaptic contacts with other cells, some of which project (send axonal output) to the same region of the spinal cord, others projecting into the brain. One target is a set of spinal interneurons that project to motor neurons controlling the arm muscles. The interneurons excite the motor neurons, and if the excitation is strong enough, some of the motor neurons generate action potentials, which travel down their axons to the point where they make excitatory synaptic contacts with muscle cells. The excitatory signals induce contraction of the muscle cells, which causes the joint angles in the arm to change, pulling the arm away.

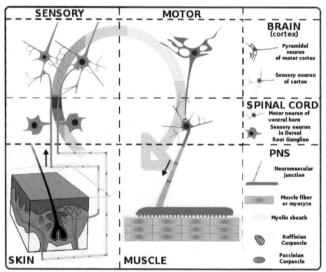

Simplified schema of basic nervous system function: signals are picked up by sensory receptors and sent to the spinal cord and brain, where processing occurs that results in signals sent back to the spinal cord and then out to motor neurons

In reality, this straightforward schema is subject to numerous complications. Although for the simplest reflexes there are short neural paths from sensory neuron to motor neuron, there are also other nearby neurons that participate in the circuit and modulate the response. Furthermore, there are projections from the brain to the spinal cord that are capable of enhancing or inhibiting the reflex.

Although the simplest reflexes may be mediated by circuits lying entirely within the spinal cord, more complex responses rely on signal processing in the brain. For example, when an object in the periphery of the visual field moves, and a person looks toward it many stages of signal processing are initiated. The initial sensory response, in the retina of the eye, and the final motor response, in the oculomotor nuclei of the brain stem, are not all that different from those in a simple reflex, but the intermediate stages are completely different. Instead of a one or two step chain of processing, the visual signals pass through perhaps a dozen stages of integration, involving the thalamus, cerebral cortex, basal ganglia, superior colliculus, cerebellum, and several brainstem nuclei. These areas perform signal-processing functions that include feature detection, perceptual analysis, memory recall, decision-making, and motor planning.

Feature detection is the ability to extract biologically relevant information from combinations of sensory signals. In the visual system, for example, sensory receptors in the retina of the eye are only individually capable of detecting "points of light" in the outside world. Second-level visual neurons receive input from groups of primary receptors, higher-level neurons receive input from groups of second-level neurons, and so on, forming a hierarchy of processing stages. At each stage, important information is extracted from the signal ensemble and unimportant information is discarded. By the end of the process, input signals representing "points of light" have been transformed into a neural representation of objects in the surrounding world and their properties. The most sophisticated sensory processing occurs inside the brain, but complex feature extraction also takes place in the spinal cord and in peripheral sensory organs such as the retina.

Intrinsic Pattern Generation

Although stimulus-response mechanisms are the easiest to understand, the nervous system is also capable of controlling the body in ways that do not require an external stimulus, by means of internally generated rhythms of activity. Because of the variety of voltage-sensitive ion channels that can be embedded in the membrane of a neuron, many types of neurons are capable, even in isolation, of generating rhythmic sequences of action potentials, or rhythmic alternations between high-rate bursting and quiescence. When neurons that are intrinsically rhythmic are connected to each other by excitatory or inhibitory synapses, the resulting networks are capable of a wide variety of dynamical behaviors, including attractor dynamics, periodicity, and even chaos. A network of neurons that uses its internal structure to generate temporally structured output, without requiring a corresponding temporally structured stimulus, is called a central pattern generator.

Internal pattern generation operates on a wide range of time scales, from milliseconds to hours or longer. One of the most important types of temporal pattern is circadian rhythmicity—that is, rhythmicity with a period of approximately 24 hours. All animals that have been studied show circadian fluctuations in neural activity, which control circadian alternations in behavior such as the sleep-wake cycle. Experimental studies dating from the 1990s have shown that circadian rhythms are generated by a "genetic clock" consisting of a special set of genes whose expression level rises and falls over the course of the day. Animals as diverse as insects and vertebrates share a similar genetic clock system. The circadian clock is influenced by light but continues to operate even when light levels are held constant and no other external time-of-day cues are available. The clock genes are expressed in many parts of the nervous system as well as many peripheral organs, but in mammals, all of these "tissue clocks" are kept in synchrony by signals that emanate from a master timekeeper in a tiny part of the brain called the suprachiasmatic nucleus.

Mirror Neurons

A mirror neuron is a neuron that fires both when an animal acts and when the animal observes the same action performed by another. Thus, the neuron "mirrors" the behavior of the other, as though the observer were itself acting. Such neurons have been directly observed in primate species. Birds have been shown to have imitative resonance behaviors and neurological evidence suggests the presence of some form of mirroring system. In humans, brain activity consistent with that of mirror neurons has been found in the premotor cortex, the supplementary motor area, the primary somatosensory cortex and the inferior parietal cortex. The function of the mirror system is a subject of much speculation. Many researchers in cognitive neuroscience and cognitive psychology consider that this system provides the physiological mechanism for the perception/action coupling. They argue that mirror neurons may be important for understanding the actions of other people, and for learning new skills by imitation. Some researchers also speculate that mirror systems may simulate observed actions, and thus contribute to theory of mind skills, while others relate mirror neurons to language abilities. However, to date, no widely accepted neural or computational models have been put forward to describe how mirror neuron activity supports cognitive functions such as imitation. There are neuroscientists who caution that the claims being made for the role of mirror neurons are not supported by adequate research.

Development

In vertebrates, landmarks of embryonic neural development include the birth and differentiation of neurons from stem cell precursors, the migration of immature neurons from their birthplaces in the embryo to their final positions, outgrowth of axons from neurons and guidance of the motile growth cone through the embryo towards postsynaptic partners, the generation of synapses between these axons and their postsynaptic partners, and finally the lifelong changes in synapses which are thought to underlie learning and memory.

All bilaterian animals at an early stage of development form a gastrula, which is polarized, with one end called the animal pole and the other the vegetal pole. The gastrula has the shape of a disk with three layers of cells, an inner layer called the endoderm, which gives rise to the lining of most internal organs, a middle layer called the mesoderm, which gives rise to the bones and muscles, and an outer layer called the ectoderm, which gives rise to the skin and nervous system.

In vertebrates, the first sign of the nervous system is the appearance of a thin strip of cells along the center of the back, called the neural plate. The inner portion of the neural plate (along the midline) is destined to become the central nervous system (CNS), the outer portion the peripheral nervous system (PNS). As development proceeds, a fold called the neural groove appears along the midline. This fold deepens, and then closes up at the top. At this point the future CNS appears as a cylindrical structure called the neural tube, whereas the future PNS appears as two strips of tissue called the neural crest, running lengthwise above the neural tube. The sequence of stages from neural plate to neural tube and neural crest is known as neurulation.

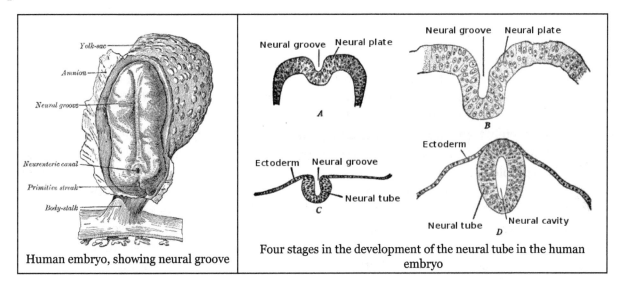

| Human embryo, showing neural groove | Four stages in the development of the neural tube in the human embryo |

In the early 20th century, a set of famous experiments by Hans Spemann and Hilde Mangold showed that the formation of nervous tissue is "induced" by signals from a group of mesodermal cells called the *organizer region*. For decades, though, the nature of the induction process defeated every attempt to figure it out, until finally it was resolved by genetic approaches in the 1990s. Induction of neural tissue requires inhibition of the gene for a so-called bone morphogenetic protein, or BMP. Specifically the protein BMP4 appears to be involved. Two proteins called Noggin and Chordin, both secreted by the mesoderm, are capable of inhibiting BMP4 and thereby inducing ectoderm to turn into neural tissue. It appears that a similar molecular mechanism is involved for widely disparate types of animals, including arthropods as well as vertebrates. In some animals, however, another type of molecule called Fibroblast Growth Factor or FGF may also play an important role in induction.

Induction of neural tissues causes formation of neural precursor cells, called neuroblasts. In drosophila, neuroblasts divide asymmetrically, so that one product is a "ganglion mother cell" (GMC), and the other is a neuroblast. A GMC divides once, to give rise to either a pair of neurons or a pair of glial cells. In all, a neuroblast is capable of generating an indefinite number of neurons or glia.

As shown in a 2008 study, one factor common to all bilateral organisms (including humans) is a family of secreted signaling molecules called neurotrophins which regulate the growth and survival of neurons. Zhu et al. identified DNT1, the first neurotrophin found in flies. DNT1 shares structural similarity with all known neurotrophins and is a key factor in the fate of neurons in Drosophila. Because neurotrophins have now been identified in both vertebrate and invertebrates, this evidence suggests that neurotrophins were present in an ancestor common to bilateral organisms and may represent a common mechanism for nervous system formation.

Pathology

The central nervous system is protected by major physical and chemical barriers. Physically, the brain and spinal cord are surrounded by tough meningeal membranes, and enclosed in the bones of the skull and spinal vertebrae, which combine to form a strong physical shield. Chemically, the brain and spinal cord are isolated by the so-called blood–brain barrier, which prevents most types of chemicals from moving from the bloodstream into the interior of the CNS. These protections make the CNS less susceptible in many ways than the PNS; the flip side, however, is that damage to the CNS tends to have more serious consequences.

Although nerves tend to lie deep under the skin except in a few places such as the ulnar nerve near the elbow joint, they are still relatively exposed to physical damage, which can cause pain, loss of sensation, or loss of muscle control. Damage to nerves can also be caused by swelling or bruises at places where a nerve passes through a tight bony channel, as happens in carpal tunnel syndrome. If a nerve is completely transected, it will often regenerate, but for long nerves this process may take months to complete. In addition to physical damage, peripheral neuropathy may be caused by many other medical problems, including genetic conditions, metabolic conditions such as diabetes, inflammatory conditions such as Guillain–Barré syndrome, vitamin deficiency, infectious diseases such as leprosy or shingles, or poisoning by toxins such as heavy metals. Many cases have no cause that can be identified, and are referred to as idiopathic. It is also possible for nerves to lose function temporarily, resulting in numbness as stiffness—common causes include mechanical pressure, a drop in temperature, or chemical interactions with local anesthetic drugs such as lidocaine.

Physical damage to the spinal cord may result in loss of sensation or movement. If an injury to the spine produces nothing worse than swelling, the symptoms may be transient, but if nerve fibers in the spine are actually destroyed, the loss of function is usually permanent. Experimental studies have shown that spinal nerve fibers attempt to regrow in the same way as nerve fibers, but in the spinal cord, tissue destruction usually produces scar tissue that cannot be penetrated by the regrowing nerves.

Organization of the Nervous System: An Overview

The nervous system can be broadly classified into two major categories – the Central Nervous System (CNS) and Peripheral Nervous System (PNS).

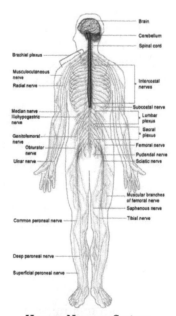

Human Nervous System

Central Nervous System

The central nervous system consists of the brain and spinal cord.

o   Brain

The brain consists of the cerebrum, cerebellum and brain stem (containing the midbrain, pons and medulla oblongata).

o   Spinal Cord

The spinal cord is a long, thin, tubular bundle of nervous tissue and support cells that extends from the brain (the medulla oblongata specifically). The brain and spinal cord together make up the central nervous system (CNS).

Peripheral Nervous System

The peripheral nervous system is divided into two parts – the somatic nervous system and the autonomic nervous system.

o   Somatic Nervous System

The somatic nervous system performs two major functions – sensory and motor. The sensory nerves innervate skin, muscles and joints, and provide information about muscle and limb position, etc. It is majorly composed of 12 cranial nerves and 33 spinal nerves.

o   Autonomic Nervous System

The autonomic nervous system can be classified into two major parts – the sympathetic and parasympathetic nervous systems. The sympathetic system participates in the body's reaction to stress, and helps in reacting to an emergency ("fight or flight") situation. The parasympathetic system conserves body resources and maintains homeostasis. About 75% of all parasympathetic nerve fibres are in the vagus nerve.

Example – Sympathetic nerves control the sudden increase in heart rate during a stressful situation, whereas the parasympathetic nerves participate in lowering the heart rate during rest.

A third part of the autonomic nervous system, called the enteric system, specifically controls the smooth muscles in the intestine.

Nerves

A nerve is an enclosed, cable-like bundle of axons (the long, slender projections of neurons) in the peripheral nervous system. A nerve provides a common pathway for the electrochemical nerve impulses that are transmitted along each of the axons.

There are three major types of nerves –

- Afferent nerves conduct signals from sensory neurons to the central nervous system, for example from the mechanoreceptors in skin.

- Efferent nerves conduct signals from the central nervous system along motor neurons to their target muscles and glands.

- Mixed nerves contain both afferent and efferent axons, and thus conduct both incoming sensory information and outgoing muscle commands in the same bundle.

Nerve fibres may also be classified into various categories based on the speed at which they conduct electrical impulses.

- Type A – Large, myelinated fibres (~120 m/s conduction velocity)

- Type C – Small, unmyelinated fibres (~0.5 m/s)

Myelin sheath – A sheath which may cover nerve fibres; it helps in faster conduction of electrical impulses.

Central Nervous System – Details

Cerebrum

The cerebrum consists of two hemispheres, joined by a large bundle of axons called the corpus callosum. The hemispheres are also connected by a smaller bundle of fibres called the anterior commisure.

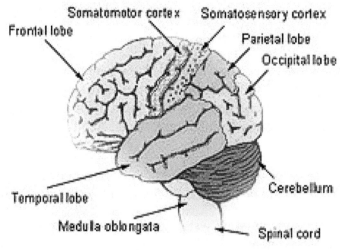

Lobes of the cerebrum.

The cerebrum can be broadly classified into four lobes –

- Frontal lobe - The frontal lobe is in the front of each cerebral hemisphere. It is separated from the parietal lobe by a vertical gap called central sulcus, and from the temporal lobe by a deep fold called the lateral (Sylvian) sulcus. Primary motor cortex, which controls voluntary movements of the body is located in the precentral gyrus, forming the posterior border of the frontal lobe. Prefrontal cortex - The prefrontal cortex (P.F.C.) is the anterior part of the frontal lobes of the brain, lying in front of the motor and premotor areas.

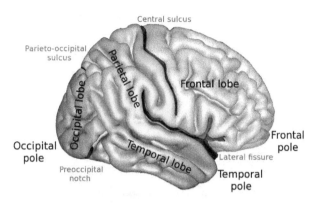

Lobes of the cerebrum.

o   "This brain region has been implicated in planning complex cognitive behavior, personality expression, decision making and moderating social behavior – a whole range of activities that are summarily described as executive function."

- Parietal Lobe - The parietal lobe is above the occipital lobe and behind the frontal lobe. It consists of the somatosensory cortex located at the anterior extreme, in the postcentral gyrus. The somatosensory cortex processes touch information coming from mechanoreceptors located in the skin, muscles and joints.

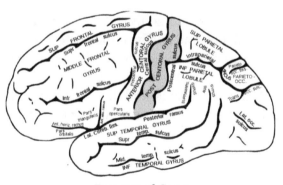

Post central Gyrus

Inferior parietal lobe consists of areas that process higher aspects of vision like spatial sense.

By virtue of its strategic location amidst three primary sensory cortices – somatosensory cortex, visual cortex and auditory cortex, - inferior parietal lobe as sensory association areas which integrate information from the three sensory modalities and extract abstract concepts.

- Temporal Lobe – The temporal lobe is located beneath the Sylvian fissure, a shared border between the temporal and frontal lobes.

Primary auditory cortex, involved in auditory processing, is located in the superior part of temporal lobe, bordering on the sylvian fissure.

The temporal lobe contains a deep structure called hippocampus, whose functions include spatial navigation, declarative memory, and memory consolidation.

Wernicke's area, which spans the region between temporal and parietal lobes, plays a key role, in language understanding, while Broca's area, which is in the frontal lobe, is responsible for language production.

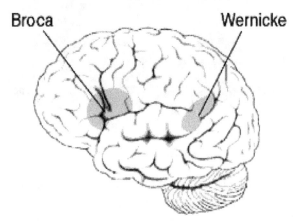

Lobes of the cerebrum.

The inferior part of temporal lobe has cortical areas that are responsible for recognizing complex visual objects, like for example, faces.

- Occipital Lobe – The occipital lobe has primary and higher areas of the visual cortex.

  o "The primary visual cortex is commonly called V1 (visual one). It is partly located in the medial side of occipital lobe and partly in the posterior pole of the occipital lobel. V1 is often also called striate cortex because it can be identified by a large stripe of myelin, the Stria of Gennari. Visually driven regions outside V1 are called extrastriate cortex. There are many extrastriate regions, and these are specialized for different visual tasks, such as visuospatial processing, color discrimination and motion perception."

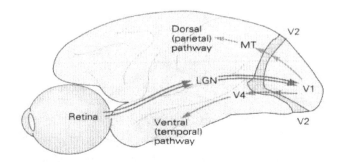

The Striate cortex

  o "Secondary and higher visual cortical areas extend from the occipital lobe and are spread over the neighboring parietal lobe."

Deep Brain Structures

- Hypothalamus - The hypothalamus is an important structure controlling our autonomous function. It links the nervous system to the endocrine system via the pituitary gland. The hypothalamus controls body temperature, hunger, thirst, fatigue, sleep, and circadian cycles.

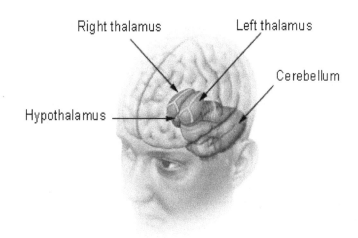

Thalamus and Hypothalamus

- Thalamus – The thalamus is located between the cerebral cortex and midbrain. It is an important hub through which most sensory information reaches the sensory cortex. It is involved in regulation of consciousness, sleep, and alertness.

- Reticular Activating System - The reticular activating system (RAS) is an area of the brain responsible for regulating arousal and sleep-wake transitions.

- Limbic System - The limbic system is a set of brain structures involved in processing emotions, and is closely related to autonomous function. This system includes the hippocampus, amygdala, anterior thalamic nuclei, septum, limbic cortex and fornix.

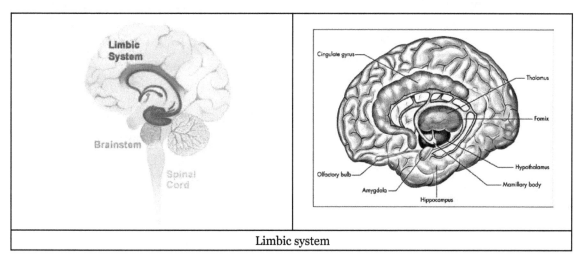

Limbic system

- Amygdala – This almond-shaped structure is located bilaterally in the medial temporal lobes of the brain. A part of the limbic system, this structure is involved in fear conditioning.

- Basal Ganglia - The basal ganglia (or basal nuclei) are a deep brain circuit consisting of 6 or 7 nuclei. This circuit receives inputs from the cortex and projects back to the cortex. It has key functions like reward processing, action selection, working memory etc

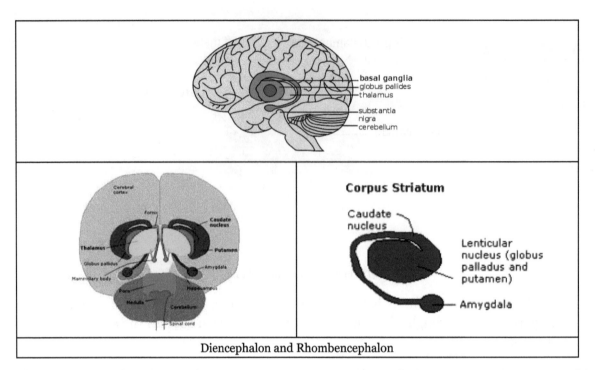

Diencephalon and Rhombencephalon

Damage to the basal ganglia can be associated to neurological and neuropsychiatric disorders like, for example, Parkinson's disease.

The following section will discuss the brain stem and cerebellum–

- Brain Stem – The brain stem is a sort of a bridge area between the cerebrum and the spinal cord. It comprises of three regions: midbrain, medulla oblongata and pons. It consists of a lot of important control centers and anatomical features. Centers for controlling cardiac and respiratory function; for regulating sleep and arousal; for controlling eating and drinking are located here.

- Medulla – This structure is a direct rostral ("towards nose") extension of the spinal cord. Its primary functions include: regulation of blood pressure and respiration.

- Pons - The pons is a a part of the brain stem, located below the midbrain and above medulla oblongata. It consists of wiring that carries: 1) motor signals from the cerebrum down to the cerebellum and medulla, and 2) sensory signals from the body into the thalamus.

- Cerebellum - The cerebellum (Latin for little brain) is a distinct structure located posteriorly under the hemispheres. It is generally thought of as a motor control unit, though its role in cognitive and affective function is well-established. It is involved in control of fine movement, equilibrium, posture, and motor learning.

- Spinal Cord - The spinal cord is a long, tail-like bundle of nerve fibers that extends from the brain (the medulla oblongata specifically) along the spine. It has three key functions:

  o Carrying motor signals from the brain to the muscle

  o Carrying sensory information in the reverse direction

  o Coordinating reflexes

Mathematical Concepts Applicable to Neurons

Eigenvalue & Eigenvectors

- A is a square matrix

$$A \in R^{n \times n} \tag{1}$$

$$AX = \lambda X \quad X \in C^n \text{ (n – Dimensional complex vector)}$$

$$\det(A - \lambda I) = 0$$

Let A be a real symmetric matrix

$$A^T = A \tag{2}$$

Or

Hermitian matrix

$$A^* = A \tag{3}$$

Theorem 1:

The Eigen values of a hermitian matrix λ_j are real.

Proof:

$$AX = \lambda X$$

$$X^T AX = \lambda X^T X$$

$$X^T AX = \lambda \|X\|^2$$

$$X^* AX = \lambda^* \|X\|^2$$

$$\lambda \|X\|^2 = \lambda^* \|X\|^2$$

λ is real

- A is skew-symmetric

$$A^T = -A \tag{4}$$

Or

$$A^* = -A$$

- $AX = \lambda X$ $\tag{5}$

$$X^T A X = \lambda X^T X$$

$$X^T A X = \lambda \|X\|^2$$

Tranposing both sides,

$$X^T A^T X = \lambda^* \|X\|^2$$

$$-X^T A X = \lambda^* \|X\|^2$$

$$\lambda \|X\|^2 = -\lambda^* \|X\|^2$$

$$\lambda = -\lambda^*$$

λ is purely imaginary.

- Q is an orthogonal matrix.

$$Q^T Q = Q Q^T = I \qquad (6)$$

Then,

$$|\lambda| = 1 \qquad (7)$$

Proof:

$$Q X = \lambda X$$

$$X^T Q^T = \lambda^* X^T$$

$$X^T Q^T Q X = \lambda \lambda^* X X^T$$

$$X^T X = \lambda \lambda^* X X^T$$

$$\|X\|^2 = |\lambda| \|X\|^2$$

$$|\lambda|^2 = 1$$

$$\lambda = e^{i\theta}$$

- For every symmetric matrix, A, then exists on orthogonal matrix, Q, such that

$$Q^T A Q = diag\left(\lambda_1, \lambda_2, \lambda_3, \dots \lambda_n\right) \qquad (8)$$

Where, $\lambda_1, \lambda_2, \lambda_3, \dots \lambda_n$ are eigenvalues of A.

Proof:

Let q_i be the eigenvector corresponding to λ_i

$$Aq_i = \lambda_i q_i$$

Let D be a matrix such that,

$$D_{ij} = q_j A q_i$$

$$D_{ij} = q_j \lambda_i q_i$$

$$if \begin{cases} i = j & \lambda_i \\ otherwise & 0 \end{cases}$$

$$Q = \left[q_1, q_2, q_3, \ldots q_n \right]_{n \times n}$$

$$Q^T A Q = D$$

$$A = QDQ^T$$

$A = \sum_{i=1}^{n} \lambda_i q_i q_i^T$ is called the eigen-decomposition of A.

- Orthogonal transformation preserves lengths:

Proof:

$$Y = QX$$

$$Y^T Y = X^T Q^T Q X$$

$$\|Y\|^2 = \|X\|^2 \tag{9}$$

Length of X equals length of Y.

Quadratic forms

Quadratic forms: Explanation

A quadratic form is a quadratic function associated with a symmetric matrix, A, and is expressed as:

$$E = X^T AX \tag{10}$$

A discussion of quadratic forms is relevant to study of neural systems since often it is required to minimize an "error function" that depends on a large number of parameters. To be able to do so, we must first define the minimum of a multivariate function. For a univariate function, f, the minimum is simply a point where f'=0 and f''>0. To define the minimum of a multivariate function, the concepts of f' and f'' must be generalized to multivariate functions.

For a multivariate function:

First derivative is the Gradient., $G = \nabla f$

Second derivative is the Hessian, H, is defined as,

$$H_{ij} = \frac{\partial^2 f}{\partial x_i \partial x_j} \tag{11}$$

Since H is a matrix and not a scalar like f', we need to specify how to define a minimum in terms of the Hessian H. It is here that we need quadratic forms. To understand this let us expand a multivariate function as a Taylor series:

$$f(X_0 + h) = f(X_0) + h^T G + \frac{1}{2!} h^T H h + \dots \text{(higher order terms)} \tag{12}$$

$f(X_0)$ is a constant and therefore does not affect the shape of $f(X)$ around X_0

Since G = 0, we may ignore the linear term $h^T G$.

The higher order terms beyond quadratic are too small and may be ignored.

Therefore, the function $f(X)$ has a minimum at X_0, if the function $\frac{1}{2!} h^T H h$

has a minimum at h = 0. To verify this, we need to examine the shape of a quadratic function $X^T A X$ around the origin (X=0).

It is easier to examine the shape of a quadratic function, in transformed coordinates, Y, obtained by rotating the original coordinates X, so that in the new coordinates the "cross-terms" are eliminated.

Geometric Interpretation of Eigenvalues in terms of Quadratic forms

For a real, symmetric matrix, A, let $Q^T A Q = D$,   (13)

where D is a diagonal matrix of eigenvalues.

Let $X = Qy$

$$E = y^T Q^T A Q y = y^T D y$$

$$E = \sum_i y_i^2 \lambda_i$$

Or,

$$\frac{\partial^2 E}{\partial y_i^2} = 2\lambda_i \tag{14}$$

Thus in the rotated coordinates, eigenvalues of A are proportional to the second derivatives of E.

Maximize the quadratic form, E, subject to $\|X\| = 1$

This can be done using the method of Lagrangian multipliers as follows. Since there is only one constraint, the Lagrange function may be written as:

$$E' = \frac{1}{2} X^T A X - \lambda (X^T X - 1)$$

$$\nabla E' = 0$$

$$\nabla E' = A X - \lambda X$$

$$A X = \lambda X$$

$$X = q_i$$

That is, the directions along which E is stationary (derivative is 0) under the constraint of $\|X\| = 1$, correspond to the eigenvectors of the matrix A, to which the quadratic form is associated.

Thus we can see that the shape of a quadratic form at the origin depends on the composition of the eigenvalues of A. Here we come to the notion of definiteness. There are 5 kinds of definiteness.

1. Positive definite: An 'n x n' matrix 'A' is said to be positive definite if it meets the following condition:

$$\frac{1}{2} X^T A X > 0, \ \forall \, X \neq 0, X \in R^n \qquad (15)$$

This implies $\lambda_i > 0$.

This case corresponds to the "minimum." Thus a multivariate function has a minimum at a point X_0, if the Hessian of the function at X_0, is positive definite.

2. Positive semi-definite: An 'n x n' matrix 'A' is said to be positive semi-definite if it meets the following condition:

$$\frac{1}{2} X^T A X \geq 0, \ \forall \, X \neq 0, X \in R^n \qquad (16)$$

This implies $\lambda_i \geq 0$

3. Negative definite: An 'n x n' matrix 'A' is said to be negative definite if it   meets the following condition:

$$\frac{1}{2} X^T A X < 0, \forall \, X \neq 0, X \in R^n \qquad (17)$$

This implies $\lambda_i < 0$

This case corresponds to the "maximum." Thus a multivariate function has a minimum at a point X_0, if the Hessian of the function at X_0, is negative definite.

4. Negative semi-definite: An 'n x n' matrix 'A' is said to be negative semi-definite if it meets the following condition:

$$\frac{1}{2}X^T AX < 0, \forall\, X \neq 0, X \in R^n \tag{18}$$

This implies $\lambda_i < 0$

5. Indefinite: An 'n x n' matrix 'A' is said to be indefinite if it does not meet any of the above four conditions.

Illustrations of various kinds of definiteness for two-variable functions.

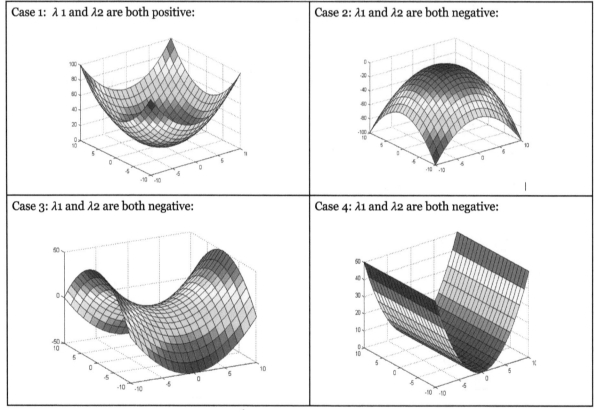

| Case 1: λ_1 and λ_2 are both positive: | Case 2: λ_1 and λ_2 are both negative: |
| Case 3: λ_1 and λ_2 are both negative: | Case 4: λ_1 and λ_2 are both negative: |

Example: For n=2, $X \in R^2, \frac{1}{2}(\lambda_1 y_1^2 + \lambda_2 y_2^2)$, plot z for all possible values of λ

Solution of linear equations: AX=b

Where, $A \in R^{n*m}, b \in R^n, X \in R^m$

Case 1

If n=m (Unique solution)

Let A^{-1} exist.

$$X = A^{-1}B \tag{19}$$

Case 2

(Least squares solution)

If n>m (Under-determined case: more equations than unknowns)

Since there may not be a perfect solution, we attempt a Least Squares solution, by minimizing E.

$E = (b - AX)^T (b - AX)$. Minimizing E gives the following solution,

$$X_{LS} = (A^T A)^{-1} A^T b = A^+ b \qquad (20)$$

Where A^+ is called the pseudo inverse. Since $b = AX_{LS} = A(A^T A)^{-1} A^T b = AA^+ b$

Case 3

m>n (Infinite solutions)

Add minimum norm condition.

$Min(\|x\|^2)$ such that Ax = b. $\qquad (21)$

Example Problem

$E = x^2 + y^2$, constraint $ax + by = c$

Let us use the method of Lagrangian Multipliers

$$E' = x^2 + y^2 + \lambda(ax + by - c)$$

$$\frac{\partial E'}{\partial x} = 2x + a\lambda = 0$$

$$\frac{\partial E'}{\partial y} = 2y + b\lambda = 0$$

$$x = -a\lambda / 2, y = -b\lambda / 2$$

$$\lambda = \frac{-2c}{a^2 + b^2}$$

$$x = \frac{ac}{a^2 + b^2}$$

$$y = \frac{bc}{a^2 + b^2}$$

$$E = X^T X$$

$$E' = X^T X - \wedge^T (AX - b)$$

$$\partial E' = 2X - (\wedge^T A)^T = 0$$

$$X = A^T \wedge /2$$

Since AX=b

$$\frac{1}{2} AA^T \wedge - b = 0$$

$$\wedge = (AA^T)^{-1} b$$

$$X = A^T (AA^T)^{-1} b$$

Dynamic Systems and Fixed Points

Dynamical Systems

Concepts from dynamic systems are most essential to study neural models. Ideas of stability, attractors, limit cycles, chaos appear again and again in discussions of brain dynamics. A few examples:

1. Memories in the brain are often modeled as attractors of brain dynamics.

2. The resting state of a neuron is considered as stable node, since the neuron returns to that state on small perturbations.

3. Periodic spiking activity of a neuron is modeled as a limit cycle.

A general dynamic system is defined as:

$$\frac{dx}{dt} = f(x), \quad x \in R^n \tag{22}$$

Stationary Points (also called, critical points, equilibrium points etc) are those where:

$$\frac{dx}{dt} = 0 = f(x), \quad at \ x = x_s \tag{23}$$

The behavior of the system around x_s, depends on the Jacobian of $f(x)$

$$A_{ij} = \frac{\partial f_i(x)}{\partial x_j} \tag{24}$$

If you linearize (22) around $x = x_s$,

$$\frac{dx}{dt} = Ax \tag{25}$$

$$\dot{x} = Ax$$

$$\dot{x}_1 = a_{11}x_1 + a_{12}x_2 + a_{13}x_3 + \ldots$$

$$\dot{x}_2 = a_{21}x_1 + a_{22}x_2 + a_{23}x_3 + \ldots$$

$$\dot{x}_3 = a_{31}x_1 + a_{32}x_2 + a_{33}x_3 + \ldots$$

Hence

$$\dot{x}_n = a_{n1}x_1 + a_{n2}x_2 + a_{n3}x_3 + \ldots + a_{nn}x_n$$

Whose solution would be,

$$X(t) = c_1 e^{\lambda_1 t} q_1 + c_2 e^{\lambda_2 t} q_2 + \ldots \tag{26}$$

Verifying:

$$\dot{x}(t) = \sum c_i \lambda_i e^{\lambda_i t} q_i$$

$$= \sum c_i e^{\lambda_i t} A q_i$$

$$= A \sum c_i e^{\lambda_i t} q_i$$

$$= Ax(t)$$

Types of stationary points (n = 2):

Description in terms of eigenvalues of A,

(Plots generated in Matlab using quiver function):

1. Both eigenvalues are real, -ve

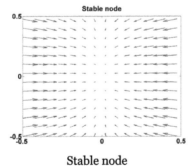

Stable node

2. Both eigenvalues real, +ve.

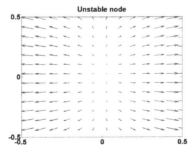

Unstable node

3. One +ve eigenvalue, one −ve eigenvalue

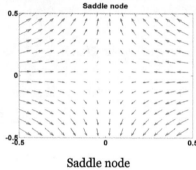

Saddle node

4. Both eigenvalues complex with −ve real parts.

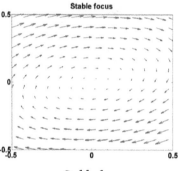

Stable focus

5. Both eigenvalues complex, +ve real parts.

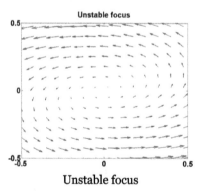

Unstable focus

6. Purely imaginary.

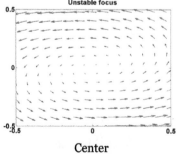

Center

Other cases:

7. Star: Both the eigenvalues being real, equal, negative

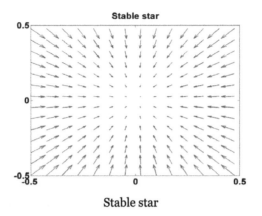

Stable star

8. One of the eigenvalues is zero.

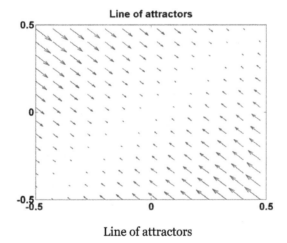

Line of attractors

Classification of Fixed Points

For a linear dynamic system,

$$\dot{x} = Ax \tag{27}$$

the type of fixed point at the origin can be related to the trace and determinant of A.

This relationship can be easily derived when A is a 2 X 2 matrix, but the result applies to the general n X n matrix.

Let

$A = \begin{bmatrix} a & b \\ c & d \end{bmatrix}$ The characteristic equation is,

$$\det\begin{pmatrix} a-\lambda & b \\ c & d-\lambda \end{pmatrix} = 0 \tag{28}$$

Expanding the determinant, we get the following quadratic equation

$$\lambda^2 - \tau\lambda + \Delta = 0 \tag{29}$$

Where

$$\tau \equiv trace(A) = a + d$$

$$\Delta \equiv det(A) = ad - bc$$

Solving for λ, we have,

$$\lambda 1, \lambda 2 = \frac{\tau \pm \sqrt{\tau^2 - 4\Delta}}{2} \tag{30}$$

From the above form of the expression for the eigenvalues, λ_1, λ_2 of the Jacobian of the dynamic system, $\dot{x} = Ax$, at the origin, we can infer a few things.

Case $\lambda < 0$:

Eigenvalues are real and have opposite signs. Therefore, the fixed point is a saddle node.

Case $\lambda > 0$:

If $\tau^2 - 4\Delta > 0$, both the roots are real. Further, $\sqrt{\tau^2 - 4\Delta}$ is less than $|\tau|$ Therefore,

- if τ is positive, both the roots are positive $\rightarrow$ unstable nodes.
- if τ is negative, both the roots are negative $\rightarrow$ stable nodes.

If $\tau^2 - 4\Delta < 0$, , the roots are complex conjugates. Furthermore,

- If τ is positive, the real part of the roots is positive $\rightarrow$ unstable focus
- If τ is negative, the real part of the roots is negative $\rightarrow$ stable focus
- If τ is 0, the roots are purely imaginary $\rightarrow$ center

The above scheme of classification is summarized in the "map" shown below.

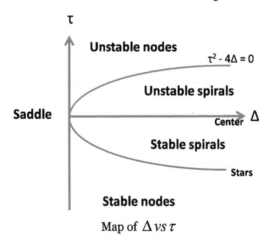

Map of Δ vs τ

Phase-plane Analysis

Above we have briefly listed out the types of fixed points that occur in a linear n-dimensional dynamic system. The origin is the only fixed point in such systems. But a nonlinear dynamic system can have multiple fixed points with a much larger repertoire of behaviors, and therefore much harder to analyze than a linear system. Therefore it is convenient to study to two-dimensional nonlinear systems which offer several advantages:

- They can be easily visualized

- They have rich dynamics and are sufficiently interesting study (for example, they exhibit limit cycle behavior, which can be used to model rhythmic behavior in real systems)

- They have a limited range of dynamics compared to n-dimensional (n>2) nonlinear dynamic systems. (for example, two-dimensional continuous, differentiable dynamic systems do not exhibit chaos).

For these reasons, two-dimensional systems occupy a special place in study of dynamic systems.

A general form of a two-dimensional dynamic system can be expressed as:

$$\dot{x} = f(x, y) \tag{31}$$

$$\dot{y} = g(x, y) \tag{32}$$

The simplest kind of analysis that can be performed on such a system is to identify all the fixed points and classify each of them by local analysis.

Fixed points of eqns. (32-33) may be calculated by solving,

$$\dot{x} = f(x, y) = 0 \tag{33}$$

$$\dot{y} = g(x, y) = 0 \tag{34}$$

Eqns (34-35) represent curves in the x-y plane and are known as null-clines.

$f(x, y) = 0$ is the x-nullcline and $g(x, y) = 0$ is the y-nullcline. The intersection points of the two null-clines are the fixed points of the system.

Let (x_0, y_0) is a fixed point of the system described by eqns. (34-35). Dynamics in the neighborhood of the fixed point may be expressed as:

$$\dot{\varepsilon}_x = f(x_0, y_0) + \varepsilon_x \frac{\partial f}{\partial x} + \varepsilon_y \frac{\partial f}{\partial y} + higher\ order\ terms \tag{35}$$

$$\dot{\varepsilon}_y = g(x_0, y_0) + \varepsilon_x \frac{\partial g}{\partial x} + \varepsilon_y \frac{\partial g}{\partial y} + higher\ order\ terms \tag{36}$$

A linear approximation of the above system is given as,

$$
\begin{bmatrix} \dot{\varepsilon}_x \\ \dot{\varepsilon}_y \end{bmatrix} = \overbrace{\begin{bmatrix} \dfrac{\partial f}{\partial x} & \dfrac{\partial f}{\partial y} \\[2mm] \dfrac{\partial g}{\partial x} & \dfrac{\partial g}{\partial y} \end{bmatrix}}^{J} \begin{bmatrix} \varepsilon_x \\ \varepsilon_y \end{bmatrix}
\tag{37}
$$

Where J denotes the Jacobian of the system eqns. (31-32)

The above equation may be expressed more compactly as,

$$
\dot{\varepsilon} = J\varepsilon
$$

The fixed point at $\varepsilon = 0$, can be classified by performing eigenvalue analysis of the above 2D system.

Limit Cycle

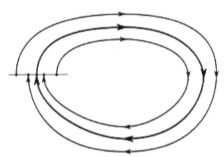

Stable limit cycle (shown in bold) and two other trajectories spiraling into it

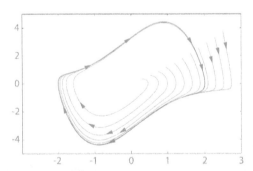

Stable limit cycle (shown in bold) for the Van der Pol oscillator

In mathematics, in the study of dynamical systems with two-dimensional phase space, a limit cycle is a closed trajectory in phase space having the property that at least one other trajectory spirals into it either as time approaches infinity or as time approaches negative infinity. Such behavior is exhibited in some nonlinear systems. Limit cycles have been used to model the behavior of a great many real world oscillatory systems. The study of limit cycles was initiated by Henri Poincaré (1854-1912).

Definition

We consider a two-dimensional dynamical system of the form

$$x'(t) = V(x(t))$$

where

$$V : \mathbb{R}^2 \to \mathbb{R}^2$$

is a smooth function. A *trajectory* of this system is some smooth function $x(t)$ with values in $\mathbb{R}^2$ which satisfies this differential equation. Such a trajectory is called *closed* (or *periodic*) if it is not constant but returns to its starting point, i.e. if there exists some $t_0 > 0$ such that $x(t + t_0) = x(t)$ for all $t \in \mathbb{R}$. An orbit is the image of a trajectory, a subset of $\mathbb{R}^2$. A *closed orbit*, or *cycle*, is the image of a closed trajectory. A *limit cycle* is a cycle which is the limit set of some other trajectory.

Properties

By the Jordan curve theorem, every closed trajectory divides the plane into two regions, the interior and the exterior of the curve.

Given a limit cycle and a trajectory in its interior that approaches the limit cycle for time approaching $+\infty$, then there is a neighborhood around the limit cycle such that *all* trajectories in the interior that start in the neighborhood approach the limit cycle for time approaching $+\infty$. The corresponding statement holds for a trajectory in the interior that approaches the limit cycle for time approaching $-\infty$, and also for trajectories in the exterior approaching the limit cycle.

Stable, Unstable and Semi-stable Limit Cycles

In the case where all the neighbouring trajectories approach the limit cycle as time approaches infinity, it is called a *stable* or *attractive* limit cycle (ω-limit cycle). If instead all neighbouring trajectories approach it as time approaches negative infinity, then it is an *unstable* limit cycle (α-limit cycle). If there is a neighbouring trajectory which spirals into the limit cycle as time approaches infinity, and another one which spirals into it as time approaches negative infinity, then it is a *semi-stable* limit cycle. There are also limit cycles which are neither stable, unstable nor semi-stable: for instance, a neighboring trajectory may approach the limit cycle from the outside, but the inside of the limit cycle is approached by a family of other cycles (which wouldn't be limit cycles).

Stable limit cycles are examples of attractors. They imply self-sustained oscillations: the closed trajectory describes perfect periodic behavior of the system, and any small perturbation from this closed trajectory causes the system to return to it, making the system stick to the limit cycle.

Finding Limit Cycles

Every closed trajectory contains within its interior a stationary point of the system, i.e. a point p where $V(p) = 0$. The Bendixson–Dulac theorem and the Poincaré–Bendixson theorem predict the absence or existence, respectively, of limit cycles of two-dimensional nonlinear dynamical systems.

Open Problems

Finding limit cycles in general is a very difficult problem. The number of limit cycles of a polynomial differential equation in the plane is the main object of the second part of Hilbert's sixteenth problem. It is unknown, for instance, whether there is any system $x' = V(x)$ in the plane where both components of V are quadratic polynomials of the two variables, such that the system has more than 4 limit cycles.

Limit cycles are a type of oscillatory behavior characterized by two properties:

- Periodicity:

A system exhibiting limit cycle behavior is confined to a closed loop trajectory and periodically visits every point on that loop. Thus, if a system whose state variable is denoted by x(t), visits a point, a, at time, t, and if 'a' is on a limit cycle,

then x(t) = x(t+T)=a,   (38)

where T is the period of the limit cycle.

- Isolatedness

This property refers to the behavior of the system when it is slightly perturbed from the limit cycle. When a system begins at a point that is in the neighborhood of a limit cycle, it either approaches the limit cycle asymptotically, or moves away from it. In this respect, a limit cycle is different from a 'center.' In case of a center, when the system is slightly perturbed, it continues on a new periodic orbit and does not return to the previous orbit.

Limit cycles are relevant to neural dynamics because neural spiking activity may be conveniently modeled as a limit cycle.

There are several ways in which it can be proved that a system exhibits limit cycle behavior, some of which are discussed below.

1) Special systems

2) Lienard Systems

3) Poincare-Benedixson Theorem

Explanation:

1) Special systems: There is no general rule for determining if a system has limit cycle behavior. This absence of general, universal methods is characteristic of nonlinear systems. But some systems have a convenient form so that it can be easily shown that they have limit cycle behavior.

Example: We can easily show the system given below has limit cycles –

$$\dot{x} = -y + \mu x\left(1 - x^2 - y^2\right) \tag{39}$$

$$\dot{y} = -x + \mu y\left(1 - x^2 - y^2\right) \tag{40}$$

Let us rewrite the above equations in polar form by substituting:

$$x = r\cos\left(\theta\right) \tag{41}$$

$$y = r\sin\left(\theta\right) \tag{42}$$

Combining eqns. (39-40) as shown below

$$x\dot{x} + y\dot{y} = \mu\left(x^2 + y^2\right)\left(1 - x^2 - y^2\right) \tag{43}$$

and expressing the result in polar coordinates we have

$$d\left(r^2\right)/dt = \mu r^2\left(1 - r^2\right) \tag{44}$$

Or,

$$\dot{r} = \frac{\mu}{2}r\left(1 - r^2\right) \tag{45}$$

Now consider,

$$\theta = \arctan\left(y/x\right) \tag{46}$$

Differentiating both sides,

$$\dot{\theta} = \frac{1}{1 + \dfrac{y^2}{x^2}}\frac{x\dot{y} - y\dot{x}}{x^2} = \frac{x\dot{y} - y\dot{x}}{r^2} \tag{47}$$

Using eqns. (39-40) we have,

$$x\dot{y} - y\dot{x} = x^2 + y^2 = r^2 \tag{48}$$

Combining eqn. (47) and eqn. (48) we have,

$$\dot{\theta} = 1 \tag{49}$$

Thus eqns. (39-40) are re-expressed as, eqns. (45) and eqn. (49).

From eqn. (45) we can see that r approaches the stable of value 1: dr/dt is positive for r < 1, and is negative for r >1.

Thus we have a limit cycle which is a circle of unit radius and angular velocity of 1.

2) Lienard systems: This represents a slight improvement over showing limit cycles only in individual systems. Lienard systems are a general class of systems that exhibit limit cycles under certain conditions.

Liénard's equation is equivalent to the system

$$\dot{x} = y \tag{50}$$

$$\dot{y} = -g(x) - f(x)y \tag{51}$$

The following theorem states that this system has a unique, stable limit cycle under appropriate hypotheses on f and g.

Liénard'sTheorem: Suppose that (x) and $g(x)$ satisfy the following conditions :

(1) $f(x)$ and $g(x)$ are continuously differentiable for all x ;

(2) $g(-x) = -g(x)$ for all x (i.e., $g(x)$ is an odd function) ;

(3) $g(x) > 0$ for $x > 0$;

(4) $f(-x) = f(x)$ for all x (i.e., $f(x)$ is an even function) ;

(5) The odd function $F(x) = \int_0^x f(u)du$ has exactly one positive zero at $x = a$, is negative

for $0 < x < a$, is positive and nondecreasing for $x > a$, and $F(x) \to \infty$ as $x \to \infty$

Then the system (50-51) has a unique, stable limit cycle surrounding the origin in the phase plane.

3) Poincare-Benedixson Theorem:

This theorem specifies conditions in 2D systems under which limit cycle exists. It is based on the idea that in a dynamic system dx/dt = f(x), where f(x) is continuous, no two trajectories intersect. Therefore, if there is a limit cycle, then all trajectories that start from inside the limit cycle will remain confined within the limit cycle. They can never come out of the limit cycle since to come out they have to cross the limit cycle, which is disallowed.

A formal statement of Poincare-Benedixson theorem is given below.

$\dot{x} = f(x)$ represents a continuously differentiable vector field on an open set containing a region R, where R is a closed, bounded subset of the plane, which is devoid of any fixed points, and There exists a trajectory C that is "confined" in R (if it starts in R it stays in R forever). If the above conditions are satisfied, C is a closed orbit.

It is not straightforward to apply Poincare-Benedixson theorem to a given system and show presence of limit cycles. Such demonstration depends crucially on construction of a trapping region, R, such that vector field on the borders of R points inwards everywhere.

There is a theorem from Index theory that any closed orbit must enclose one or more fixed points. Since Poincare-Benedixson requires that R must not include any fixed points, we need to construct an R that excludes all fixed points. Typically a ring-like, annular region is chosen such that vector field is pointed inwards on the outer boundary, and outwards on the inner boundary. If such a region can be constructed, Poincare-Benedixson assures us that a limit cycle exists inside R. Exact construction of R depends on the details of the equations that describe the system.

Limit Cycle Generation by Bifurcation

As the parameters of a dynamic system are changed gradually, at certain critical values of the parameters, the dynamics can change qualitatively.(For example, in the map of figure, a stable focus changes into an unstable focus when we cross the Δ axis from below). Such qualitative changes in dynamics are known as bifurcations. The parameter values where such changes occurs are called bifurcation points.

The map of Figure which shows different types of fixed points on the $-\Delta$ plane is a simple example of bifurcations. The plane is divided into several regions, where each region represents one type of fixed point, or a dynamical regime. When we crossover from one region to a neighboring region, dynamics suddenly changes, and a bifurcation occurs. For example, when we cross the $\Delta - axis\,(\tau = 0\ line)$, saddle node become either stable or unstable nodes.

Four important types of bifurcations by which limit cycles can be produced are:

    a) Supercritical Andronov-Hopf bifurcation

    b) Subcritical Andronov-Hopf bifurcation

    c) Saddle-node bifurcation

    d) Saddle-node on invariant circle bifurcation

a) Andronov-Hopf Bifurcation – supercritical

In Andronov-Hopf bifurcation, a stable focus gets converted into an unstable focus giving rise to a limit cycle in the process. A stable focus has complex valued eigenvalues with negative real parts; the eigenvalues of the unstable focus has positive real parts. Thus Andronov-Hopf bifurcation occurs when a pair of complex conjugate eigenvalues cross over from the left halfplane to the right.

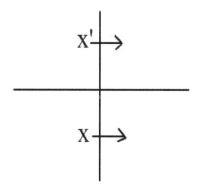

Depending on the precise manner in which a stable focus gets destabilized and leads to a limit cycle, the Andronov-Hopf bifurcation can be classified into two types.

In supercritical Andronov-Hopf bifurcation, when a stable focus becomes a limit cycle, the limit cycle first starts with a small/infinitesimal amplitude and gradually increases in size.

This behavior can be seen in an example.

Example:

$$\dot{r} = \mu r - r^3 \tag{52}$$

$$\dot{\theta} = \omega + br^2 \tag{53}$$

Note that θ does not influence evolution of r (in Eqn. 52) but r influences θ (in eqn. 53). Therefore changes in amplitude may be studied solely by studying Eqn. (52).

Note how the steady state value of r changes as μ is increased from a negative value to a positive value. For $\mu < 0$, the only real solution is r = 0; for $\mu > 0$, there are three real solutions: r = 0, +sqrt(μ). Since r has to be positive, the solutions are r = 0 and sqrt(μ). Eqn. (53) simply says that angular velocity increases with increasing radius.

Therefore, if we express the steadystate radius, r_s, as a function of bifurcation parameter μ,

$$r_s = \sqrt{\mu}, \mu > 0$$
$$\text{For } \mu > 0 \text{ and} \tag{54}$$
$$= 0, \mu \leq 0$$

It can be easily verified that in the system defined by eqns. (52-53), the eigenvalues at the origin cross over from the left half-plane to the right, as μ crosses over from negative to positive values.

Eigen Values Analysis for Eqns. (52-53)

$$\dot{x} = \dot{r}\cos\theta - r\dot{\theta}\sin\theta$$

$$= \left(\mu v - r^3\right)\cos(\theta) - r\left(\omega + br^2\right)\sin(\theta)$$

$$= \left(\mu - \left(x^2 + y^2\right)\right)x - \left(\omega + b\left(x^2 + y^2\right)\right)y$$

$$= \mu x - \omega y + cubic\,terms \tag{55}$$

$$y = r\sin\theta$$

$$\dot{y} = r\sin\theta + r\cos\theta\dot{\theta}$$

$$= \left(\mu v - r^3\right)\sin\theta + r\cos\theta\left(\omega + br^2\right)$$
$$= \left(\mu - r^2\right)y + x\left(\omega + br^2\right)$$
$$= (\mu - x^2 - y^2)y + x(\omega + b(x^2 + y^2))$$
$$= \mu y + \omega x + cubic\,terms \tag{56}$$

$$A = \begin{bmatrix} \mu - \omega \\ \omega - \mu \end{bmatrix}$$

$$\lambda = \mu \pm i\omega \qquad\qquad (57)$$

$\mu < 0$ – *stable focus*

$\mu > 0$ – *unstable focus*

Properties of Supercritical Andronov-Hopf bifurcation

Size of the limit cycle, r_0, grows as $\sqrt{\mu - \mu_c}$ for μ close to and greater than μ_c.

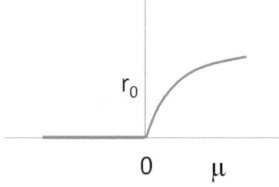

Size of the limit cycle r_0 vs μ

2.   Frequency $\approx \omega = I_m[\lambda]$, evaluated at $\mu = \mu_c$

Formula is exact at birth of the limit cycle.

$$T = \frac{L\pi}{I_m[\lambda] + \theta(\mu - \mu_c)} \qquad\qquad (58)$$

$$\dot{r} = \mu r - r^3$$
$$= r(\mu - r^2)$$

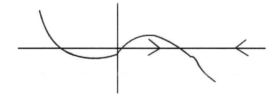

$\mu > 0$

b) Subcritical Andronov-Hopf bifurcation:-

In a subcritical Andronov-Hopf bifurcation, when the unstable focus destabilized, a limit cycle of finite size sudden appears, unlike in the supercritical case the limit cycle starts of small and grows gradually as the bifurcation parameter increases.

An example of a system which exhibits subcritical Andronov-Hopf bifurcation is given below:

$$\dot{r} = \mu r + r^3 - r^5$$
$$\dot{\theta} = \omega + br^2 \tag{59}$$

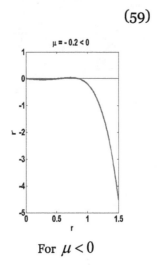

For $\mu < 0$

Thus for $\mu < 0$, there is no limit cycle; there is a stable fixed point at the origin

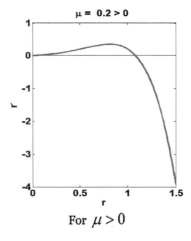

For $\mu > 0$

But when $\mu > 0$, there is suddenly a limit cycle at $r = r_0$, a finite value

Thus, in supercritical Andronov-Hopf bifurcation, the size of limit cycle varies as a function of μ as follows:

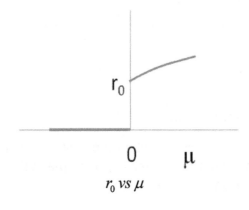

r_0 vs μ

c) Saddle Node Bifurcation of Cycles:

In saddle node bifurcation of cycles (also called a fold bifurcation), two limit cycles coalesce and annihilate each other. A simple example system that exhibits Saddle node bifurcation of cycles is,

$$\dot{r} = \mu r + r^3 - r^5$$
$$\dot{\theta} = \omega + br^2$$

Note the system is the same as the one used in case of the subcritical Andronov-Hopf bifurcation above. But the difference lies in the value of bifurcation parameter at which the bifurcation occurs.

In case of subcritical Andronov-Hopf bifurcation, the bifurcation occurred at $\mu = 0$. For $\mu < 0$, there is a stable focus at the origin, an unstable limit cycle of lesser radius, and a stable limit cycle of larger radius. When $\mu > 0$, the unstable limit cycle merges with the origin and disappears. The stable limit cycle only remains.

In case of Saddle node bifurcation of cycles, the bifurcation occurs at $\mu = -1/4$

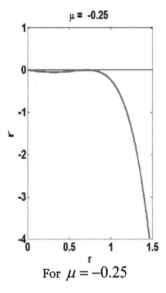

For $\mu = -0.25$

For $\mu < -1/4 \left(\mu < \mu_c \right)$, (origin is the only stable point. There are no limit cycles (stable or unstable).

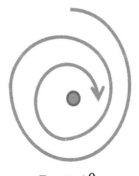

For $\mu < 0$

For $\mu\left(\mu=\mu_c\right)$,

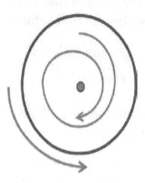

For $\mu=\mu_c$

For $\left(\mu>\mu_c\right)$: For $\mu>-1/4$, origin is still a stable point. But in addition there are now two limit cycles (one stable and the other unstable).

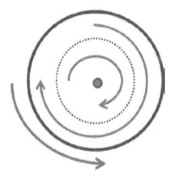

For $\mu=\mu_c$

Therefore a key difference between subcritical Andronov-Hopf bifurcation and Saddle node bifurcation of cycles is that in the former, the stable focus at the origin becomes unstable after bifurcation, whereas in the latter the focus at the origin remains stable throughout.

d) Saddle Node on Invariant Circle:

In this type of bifurcation, a node and saddle are located on a loop – the invariant circle. By varying a bifurcation parameter, the saddle and the node come together, coalesce and annihilate each other leaving the loop, the limit cycle, intact.

A sample system that displays Saddle node on invariant Circle behavior:

$$\dot{r}=r\left(1-r^2\right)$$
$$\dot{\theta}=\mu-\sin\left(\theta\right) \qquad\qquad\qquad (60)$$

For $\mu<1$, the phase dynamic equation has two solutions – saddle and a node located on the unit circle (r = 1). Phase portrait is shown in the figure below. As $\mu\rightarrow1$, the saddle and the node approach each other and coalesce. When $\mu>1$, the saddle and the node annihilate each other leaving a limit cycle at r = 1.

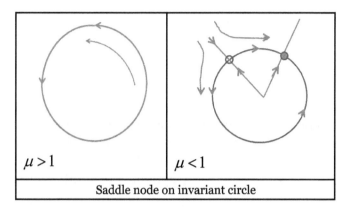

Saddle node on invariant circle

Homoclinic Bifurcation

A homoclinic orbit is one in which a trajectory starts at a saddle node, makes a loop, and returns to the same saddle node. In a homoclinic bifurcation, a closed loop approaches a saddle node. At bifurcation, the saddle touches the loop, transforming the loop into a homoclinic orbit. Thus trajectories that start from the saddle go along the loop and return to the saddle in the opposite direction.

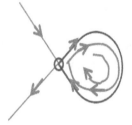

The limit cycle with the saddle outside

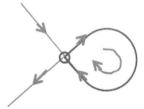

The saddle had merged with the limit cycle. The cycle has now become a homoclinic orbit

Neuroinformatics

Neuroinformatics is a research field concerned with the organization of neuroscience data by the application of computational models and analytical tools. These areas of research are important for the integration and analysis of increasingly large-volume, high-dimensional, and fine-grain experimental data. Neuroinformaticians provide computational tools, mathematical models, and create interoperable databases for clinicians and research scientists. Neuroscience is a heterogeneous field, consisting of many and various sub-disciplines (e.g., cognitive psychology, behavioral neuroscience, and behavioral genetics). In order for our understanding of the brain to continue to deepen, it is necessary that these sub-disciplines are able to share data and findings in a meaningful way; Neuroinformaticians facilitate this.

Neuroinformatics stands at the intersection of neuroscience and information science. Other fields, like genomics, have demonstrated the effectiveness of freely distributed databases and the application of theoretical and computational models for solving complex problems. In Neuroinformatics, such facilities allow researchers to more easily quantitatively confirm their working theories by computational modeling. Additionally, neuroinformatics fosters collaborative research—an important fact that facilitates the field's interest in studying the multi-level complexity of the brain.

There are three main directions where neuroinformatics has to be applied:

1. the development of tools and databases for management and sharing of neuroscience data at all levels of analysis,

2. the development of tools for analyzing and modeling neuroscience data,

3. the development of computational models of the nervous system and neural processes.

In the recent decade, as vast amounts of diverse data about the brain were gathered by many research groups, the problem was raised of how to integrate the data from thousands of publications in order to enable efficient tools for further research. The biological and neuroscience data are highly interconnected and complex, and by itself, integration represents a great challenge for scientists.

Combining informatics research and brain research provides benefits for both fields of science. On one hand, informatics facilitates brain data processing and data handling, by providing new electronic and software technologies for arranging databases, modeling and communication in brain research. On the other hand, enhanced discoveries in the field of neuroscience will invoke the development of new methods in information technologies (IT).

History

Starting in 1989, the United States National Institute of Mental Health (NIMH), the National Institute of Drug Abuse (NIDA) and the National Science Foundation (NSF) provided the National Academy of Sciences Institute of Medicine with funds to undertake a careful analysis and study of the need to create databases, share neuroscientific data and to examine how the field of information technology could create the tools needed for the increasing volume and modalities of neuroscientific data. The positive recommendations were reported in 1991 ("Mapping The Brain And Its Functions. Integrating Enabling Technologies Into Neuroscience Research." National Academy Press, Washington, D.C. ed. Pechura, C.M., and Martin, J.B.) This positive report enabled NIMH, now directed by Allan Leshner, to create the "Human Brain Project" (HBP), with the first grants awarded in 1993. The HBP was led by Koslow along with cooperative efforts of other NIH Institutes, the NSF, the National Aeronautics and Space Administration and the Department of Energy. The HPG and grant-funding initiative in this area slightly preceded the explosive expansion of the World Wide Web. From 1993 through 2004 this program grew to over 100 million dollars in funded grants.

Next, Koslow pursued the globalization of the HPG and neuroinformatics through the European Union and the Office for Economic Co-operation and Development (OECD), Paris, France. Two particular opportunities occurred in 1996.

- The first was the existence of the US/European Commission Biotechnology Task force co-chaired by Mary Clutter from NSF. Within the mandate of this committee, of which Koslow was a member the United States European Commission Committee on Neuroinformatics was established and co-chaired by Koslow from the United States. This committee resulted in the European Commission initiating support for neuroinformatics in Framework 5 and it has continued to support activities in neuroinformatics research and training.

- A second opportunity for globalization of neuroinformatics occurred when the participating governments of the Mega Science Forum (MSF) of the OECD were asked if they had any new scientific initiatives to bring forward for scientific cooperation around the globe. The White House Office of Science and Technology Policy requested that agencies in the federal government meet at NIH to decide if cooperation were needed that would be of global benefit. The NIH held a series of meetings in which proposals from different agencies were discussed. The proposal recommendation from the U.S. for the MSF was a combination of the NSF and NIH proposals. Jim Edwards of NSF supported databases and data-sharing in the area of biodiversity; Koslow proposed the HPG ? as a model for sharing neuroscientific data, with the new moniker of *neuroinformatics*.

The two related initiates were combined to form the United States proposal on "Biological Informatics". This initiative was supported by the White House Office of Science and Technology Policy and presented at the OECD MSF by Edwards and Koslow. An MSF committee was established on Biological Informatics with two subcommittees: 1. Biodiversity (Chair, James Edwards, NSF), and 2. Neuroinformatics (Chair, Stephen Koslow, NIH). At the end of two years the Neuroinformatics subcommittee of the Biological Working Group issued a report supporting a global neuroinformatics effort. Koslow, working with the NIH and the White House Office of Science and Technology Policy to establishing a new Neuroinformatics working group to develop specific recommendation to support the more general recommendations of the first report. The Global Science Forum (GSF; renamed from MSF) of the OECD supported this recommendation.

The International Neuroinformatics Coordinating Facility

This committee presented 3 recommendations to the member governments of GSF. These recommendations were:

1. National neuroinformatics programs should be continued or initiated in each country should have a national node to both provide research resources nationally and to serve as the contact for national and international coordination.

2. An International Neuroinformatics Coordinating Facility (INCF) should be established. The INCF will coordinate the implementation of a global neuroinformatics network through integration of national neuroinformatics nodes.

3. A new international funding scheme should be established. This scheme should eliminate national and disciplinary barriers and provide a most efficient approach to global collabo-

rative research and data sharing. In this new scheme, each country will be expected to fund the participating researchers from their country.

The GSF neuroinformatics committee then developed a business plan for the operation, support and establishment of the INCF which was supported and approved by the GSF Science Ministers at its 2004 meeting. In 2006 the INCF was created and its central office established and set into operation at the Karolinska Institute, Stockholm, Sweden under the leadership of Sten Grillner. Sixteen countries (Australia, Canada, China, the Czech Republic, Denmark, Finland, France, Germany, India, Italy, Japan, the Netherlands, Norway, Sweden, Switzerland, the United Kingdom and the United States), and the EU Commission established the legal basis for the INCF and Programme in International Neuroinformatics (PIN). To date, fourteen countries (Czech Republic, Finland, France, Germany, Italy, Japan, Norway, Sweden, Switzerland, and the United States) are members of the INCF. Membership is pending for several other countries.

The goal of the INCF is to coordinate and promote international activities in neuroinformatics. The INCF contributes to the development and maintenance of database and computational infrastructure and support mechanisms for neuroscience applications. The system is expected to provide access to all freely accessible human brain data and resources to the international research community. The more general task of INCF is to provide conditions for developing convenient and flexible applications for neuroscience laboratories in order to improve our knowledge about the human brain and its disorders.

Society for Neuroscience Brain Information Group

On the foundation of all of these activities, Huda Akil, the 2003 President of the Society for Neuroscience (SfN) established the Brain Information Group (BIG) to evaluate the importance of neuroinformatics to neuroscience and specifically to the SfN. Following the report from BIG, SfN also established a neuroinformatics committee.

In 2004, SfN announced the Neuroscience Database Gateway (NDG) as a universal resource for neuroscientists through which almost any neuroscience databases and tools may be reached. The NDG was established with funding from NIDA, NINDS and NIMH. The Neuroscience Database Gateway has transitioned to a new enhanced platform, the Neuroscience Information Framework. Funded by the NIH Neuroscience BLueprint, the NIF is a dynamic portal providing access to neuroscience-relevant resources (data, tools, materials) from a single search interface. The NIF builds upon the foundation of the NDG, but provides a unique set of tools tailored especially for neuroscientists: a more expansive catalog, the ability to search multiple databases directly from the NIF home page, a custom web index of neuroscience resources, and a neuroscience-focused literature search function.

Collaboration with Other Disciplines

Neuroinformatics is formed at the intersections of the following fields:

- neuroscience
- computer science
- biology

- experimental psychology

- medicine

- engineering

- physical sciences

- mathematics

- chemistry

Biology is concerned with molecular data (from genes to cell specific expression); medicine and anatomy with the structure of synapses and systems level anatomy; engineering – electrophysiology (from single channels to scalp surface EEG), brain imaging; computer science – databases, software tools, mathematical sciences – models, chemistry – neurotransmitters, etc. Neuroscience uses all aforementioned experimental and theoretical studies to learn about the brain through its various levels. Medical and biological specialists help to identify the unique cell types, and their elements and anatomical connections. Functions of complex organic molecules and structures, including a myriad of biochemical, molecular, and genetic mechanisms which regulate and control brain function, are determined by specialists in chemistry and cell biology. Brain imaging determines structural and functional information during mental and behavioral activity. Specialists in biophysics and physiology study physical processes within neural cells neuronal networks. The data from these fields of research is analyzed and arranged in databases and neural models in order to integrate various elements into a sophisticated system; this is the point where neuroinformatics meets other disciplines.

Neuroscience provides the following types of data and information on which neuroinformatics operates:

- Molecular and cellular data (ion channel, action potential, genetics, cytology of neurons, protein pathways),

- Data from organs and systems (visual cortex, perception, audition, sensory system, pain, taste, motor system, spinal cord),

- Cognitive data (language, emotion, motor learning, sexual behavior, decision making, social neuroscience),

- Developmental information (neuronal differentiation, cell survival, synaptic formation, motor differentiation, injury and regeneration, axon guidance, growth factors),

- Information about diseases and aging (autonomic nervous system, depression, anxiety, Parkinson's disease, addiction, memory loss),

- Neural engineering data (brain-computer interface), and

- Computational neuroscience data (computational models of various neuronal systems, from membrane currents, proteins to learning and memory).

Neuroinformatics uses databases, the Internet, and visualization in the storage and analysis of the mentioned neuroscience data.

Research Programs and Groups

Australia

Neuroimaging & Neuroinformatics, Howard Florey Institute, University of Melbourne

> Institute scientists utilize brain imaging techniques, such as magnetic resonance imaging, to reveal the organization of brain networks involved in human thought. Led by Gary Egan.

Denmark

The THOR Center for Neuroinformatics

> Established April 1998 at the Department of Mathematical Modelling, Technical University of Denmark. Besides pursuing independent research goals, the THOR Center hosts a number of related projects concerning neural networks, functional neuroimaging, multimedia signal processing, and biomedical signal processing.

Germany

The Neuroinformatics Portal Pilot

> The project is part of a larger effort to enhance the exchange of neuroscience data, data-analysis tools, and modeling software. The portal is supported from many members of the OECD Working Group on Neuroinformatics. The Portal Pilot is promoted by the German Ministry for Science and Education.

Computational Neuroscience, ITB, Humboldt-University Berlin

> This group focuses on computational neurobiology, in particular on the dynamics and signal processing capabilities of systems with spiking neurons. Lead by Andreas VM Herz.

The Neuroinformatics Group in Bielefeld

> Active in the field of Artificial Neural Networks since 1989. Current research programmes within the group are focused on the improvement of man-machine-interfaces, robot-force-control, eye-tracking experiments, machine vision, virtual reality and distributed systems.

Italy

Laboratory of Computational Embodied Neuroscience (LOCEN)

> This group, part of the Institute of Cognitive Sciences and Technologies, Italian National Research Council (ISTC-CNR) in Rome and founded in 2006 is currently led by Gianluca Baldassarre. It has two objectives: (a) understanding the brain mechanisms underlying learning and expression of sensorimotor behaviour, and related motivations and higher-level cognition grounded on it, on the basis of embodied computational models; (b) transferring the acquired knowledge to building innovative controllers for autonomous humanoid robots capable of learning in an open-ended fashion on the basis of intrinsic and extrinsic motivations.

Japan

Japan National Neuroinformatics Resource

The Visiome Platform is the Neuroinformatics Search Service that provides access to mathematical models, experimental data, analysis libraries and related resources. An online portal for neurophysiological data sharing is also available at BrainLiner.jp as part of the MEXT Strategic Research Program for Brain Sciences (SRPBS).

Laboratory for Mathematical Neuroscience, RIKEN Brain Science Institute (Wako, Saitama)

The target of Laboratory for Mathematical Neuroscience is to establish mathematical foundations of brain-style computations toward construction of a new type of information science. Led by Shun-ichi Amari.

The Netherlands

Netherlands state program in neuroinformatics

Started in the light of the international OECD Global Science Forum which aim is to create a worldwide program in Neuroinformatics.

Pakistan

NUST-SEECS Neuroinformatics Research Lab

Establishment of the Neuro-Informatics Lab at SEECS-NUST has enabled Pakistani researchers and members of the faculty to actively participate in such efforts, thereby becoming an active part of the above-mentioned experimentation, simulation, and visualization processes. The lab collaborates with the leading international institutions to develop highly skilled human resource in the related field. This lab facilitates neuroscientists and computer scientists in Pakistan to conduct their experiments and analysis on the data collected using state of the art research methodologies without investing in establishing the experimental neuroscience facilities. The key goal of this lab is to provide state of the art experimental and simulation facilities, to all beneficiaries including higher education institutes, medical researchers/practitioners, and technology industry.

Switzerland

The Blue Brain Project

The Blue Brain Project was founded in May 2005, and uses an 8000 processor Blue Gene/L supercomputer developed by IBM. At the time, this was one of the fastest supercomputers in the world.

The project involves:

- Databases: 3D reconstructed model neurons, synapses, synaptic pathways, microcircuit statistics, computer model neurons, virtual neurons.

- Visualization: microcircuit builder and simulation results visualizator, 2D, 3D and immersive visualization systems are being developed.

- Simulation: a simulation environment for large-scale simulations of morphologically complex neurons on 8000 processors of IBM's Blue Gene supercomputer.

- Simulations and experiments: iterations between large-scale simulations of neocortical microcircuits and experiments in order to verify the computational model and explore predictions.

The mission of the Blue Brain Project is to understand mammalian brain function and dysfunction through detailed simulations. The Blue Brain Project will invite researchers to build their own models of different brain regions in different species and at different levels of detail using Blue Brain Software for simulation on Blue Gene. These models will be deposited in an internet database from which Blue Brain software can extract and connect models together to build brain regions and begin the first whole brain simulations.

The Institute of Neuroinformatics (INI)

Established at the University of Zurich at the end of 1995, the mission of the Institute is to discover the key principles by which brains work and to implement these in artificial systems that interact intelligently with the real world.

United Kingdom

Genes to Cognition Project

> A neuroscience research programme that studies genes, the brain and behaviour in an integrated manner. It is engaged in a large-scale investigation of the function of molecules found at the synapse. This is mainly focused on proteins that interact with the NMDA receptor, a receptor for the neurotransmitter, glutamate, which is required for processes of synaptic plasticity such as long-term potentiation (LTP). Many of the techniques used are high-throughout in nature, and integrating the various data sources, along with guiding the experiments has raised numerous informatics questions. The program is primarily run by Professor Seth Grant at the Wellcome Trust Sanger Institute, but there are many other teams of collaborators across the world.

The CARMEN project

> The CARMEN project is a multi-site (11 universities in the United Kingdom) research project aimed at using GRID computing to enable experimental neuroscientists to archive their datasets in a structured database, making them widely accessible for further research, and for modellers and algorithm developers to exploit.

EBI Computational Neurobiology, EMBL-EBI (Hinxton)

> The main goal of the group is to build realistic models of neuronal function at various levels, from the synapse to the micro-circuit, based on the precise knowledge of molecule functions and interactions (Systems Biology). Led by Nicolas Le Novère.

United States

Neuroscience Information Framework

The Neuroscience Information Framework (NIF) is an initiative of the NIH Blueprint for Neuroscience Research, which was established in 2004 by the National Institutes of Health. Unlike general search engines, NIF provides deeper access to a more focused set of resources that are relevant to neuroscience, search strategies tailored to neuroscience, and access to content that is traditionally "hidden" from web search engines. The NIF is a dynamic inventory of neuroscience databases, annotated and integrated with a unified system of biomedical terminology (i.e. NeuroLex). NIF supports concept-based queries across multiple scales of biological structure and multiple levels of biological function, making it easier to search for and understand the results. NIF will also provide a registry through which resources providers can disclose availability of resources relevant to neuroscience research. NIF is not intended to be a warehouse or repository itself, but a means for disclosing and locating resources elsewhere available via the web.

Neurogenetics GeneNetwork

Genenetwork started as component of the NIH Human Brain Project in 1999 with a focus on the genetic analysis of brain structure and function. This international program consists of tightly integrated genome and phenome data sets for human, mouse, and rat that are designed specifically for large-scale systems and network studies relating gene variants to differences in mRNA and protein expression and to differences in CNS structure and behavior. The great majority of data are open access. GeneNetwork has a companion neuroimaging web site—the Mouse Brain Library—that contains high resolution images for thousands of genetically defined strains of mice.

The Neuronal Time Series Analysis (NTSA)

NTSA Workbench is a set of tools, techniques and standards designed to meet the needs of neuroscientists who work with neuronal time series data. The goal of this project is to develop information system that will make the storage, organization, retrieval, analysis and sharing of experimental and simulated neuronal data easier. The ultimate aim is to develop a set of tools, techniques and standards in order to satisfy the needs of neuroscientists who work with neuronal data.

The Cognitive Atlas

The Cognitive Atlas is a project developing a shared knowledge base in cognitive science and neuroscience. This comprises two basic kinds of knowledge: tasks and concepts, providing definitions and properties thereof, and also relationships between them. An important feature of the site is ability to cite literature for assertions (e.g. "The Stroop task measures executive control") and to discuss their validity. It contributes to NeuroLex and the Neuroscience Information Framework, allows programmatic access to the database, and is built around semantic web technologies.

Brain Big Data research group at the Allen Institute for Brain Science (Seattle, WA)

Led by Hanchuan Peng, this group has focused on using large-scale imaging computing and data analysis techniques to reconstruct single neuron models and mapping them in brains of different animals.

Technologies and Developments

The main technological tendencies in neuroinformatics are:

1. Application of computer science for building databases, tools, and networks in neuroscience;

2. Analysis and modeling of neuronal systems.

In order to organize and operate with neural data scientists need to use the standard terminology and atlases that precisely describe the brain structures and their relationships.

- Neuron Tracing and Reconstruction is an essential technique to establish digital models of the morphology of neurons. Such morphology is useful for neuron classification and simulation.

- BrainML is a system that provides a standard XML metaformat for exchanging neuroscience data.

- The Biomedical Informatics Research Network (BIRN) is an example of a grid system for neuroscience. BIRN is a geographically distributed virtual community of shared resources offering vast scope of services to advance the diagnosis and treatment of disease. BIRN allows combining databases, interfaces and tools into a single environment.

- Budapest Reference Connectome is a web-based 3D visualization tool to browse connections in the human brain. Nodes, and connections are calculated from the MRI datasets of the Human Connectome Project.

- GeneWays is concerned with cellular morphology and circuits. GeneWays is a system for automatically extracting, analyzing, visualizing and integrating molecular pathway data from the research literature. The system focuses on interactions between molecular substances and actions, providing a graphical view on the collected information and allows researchers to review and correct the integrated information.

- Neocortical Microcircuit Database (NMDB). A database of versatile brain's data from cells to complex structures. Researchers are able not only to add data to the database but also to acquire and edit one.

- SenseLab. SenseLab is a long-term effort to build integrated, multidisciplinary models of neurons and neural systems. It was founded in 1993 as part of the original Human Brain Project. A collection of multilevel neuronal databases and tools. SenseLab contains six related databases that support experimental and theoretical research on the membrane properties that mediate information processing in nerve cells, using the olfactory pathway as a model system.

- BrainMaps.org is an interactive high-resolution digital brain atlas using a high-speed database and virtual microscope that is based on over 12 million megapixels of scanned images of several species, including human.

Another approach in the area of the brain mappings is the probabilistic atlases obtained from the real data from different group of people, formed by specific factors, like age, gender, diseased etc. Provides more flexible tools for brain research and allow obtaining more reliable and precise results, which cannot be achieved with the help of traditional brain atlases.

Cellular Neuroscience

Cellular neuroscience is the study of neurons at a cellular level. This includes morphology and physiological properties of single neurons. Several techniques such as intracellular recording, patch-clamp, and voltage-clamp technique, pharmacology, confocal imaging, molecular biology, two photon laser scanning microscopy and Ca^{2+} imaging have been used to study activity at the cellular level. Cellular neuroscience examines the various types of neurons, the functions of different neurons, the influence of neurons upon each other, how neurons work together.

Neurons and Glial Cells

Neurons are cells that are specialized to receive, propagate, and transmit electrochemical impulses. In the human brain alone, there are over eighty billion neurons. Neurons are diverse with respect to morphology and function. Thus, not all neurons correspond to the stereotypical motor neuron with dendrites and myelinated axons that conduct action potentials. Some neurons such as photoreceptor cells, for example, do not have myelinated axons that conduct action potentials. Other unipolar neurons found in invertebrates do not even have distinguishing processes such as dendrites. Moreover, the distinctions based on function between neurons and other cells such as cardiac and muscle cells are not helpful. Thus, the fundamental difference between a neuron and a nonneuronal cell is a matter of degree.

Another major class of cells found in the nervous system are glial cells. These cells are only recently beginning to receive attention from neurobiologists for being involved not just in nourishment and support of neurons, but also in modulating synapses. For example, Schwann cells, which are a type of glial cell found in the peripheral nervous system, modulate synaptic connections between presynaptic terminals of motor neuron endplates and muscle fibers at neuromuscular junctions.

Neuronal Function

One prominent characteristic of many neurons is excitability. Neurons generate electrical impulses or changes in voltage of two types: graded potentials and action potentials. Graded potentials occur when the membrane potential depolarizes and hyperpolarizes in a graded fashion relative to the amount of stimulus that is applied to the neuron. An action potential on the other hand is an all-or-none electrical impulse. Despite being slower than graded potentials, action potentials have the advantage of traveling long distances in axons with little or no decrement. Much of the current knowledge of action potentials comes from squid axon experiments by Sir Alan Lloyd Hodgkin and Sir Andrew Huxley.

Action Potential

The Hodgkin–Huxley model of an action potential in the squid giant axon has been the basis for much of the current understanding of the ionic bases of action potentials. Briefly, the model states that the generation of an action potential is determined by two ions: Na+ and K+. An action potential can be divided into several sequential phases: threshold, rising phase, falling phase, undershoot phase, and recovery. Following several local graded depolarizations of the membrane potential, the threshold of excitation is reached, voltage-gated sodium channels are activated, which leads to an influx of Na+ ions. As Na+ ions enter the cell, the membrane potential is further depolarized, and more voltage-gated sodium channels are activated. Such a process is also known as a positive feedback loop. As the rising phase reaches its peak, voltage-gated Na+ channels are inactivated whereas voltage-gated K+ channels are activated, resulting in a net outward movement of K+ ions, which repolarizes the membrane potential towards the resting membrane potential. Repolarization of the membrane potential continues, resulting in an undershoot phase or absolute refractory period. The undershoot phase occurs because unlike voltage-gated sodium channels, voltage-gated potassium channels inactivate much more slowly. Nevertheless, as more voltage-gated K+ channels become inactivated, the membrane potential recovers to its normal resting steady state..

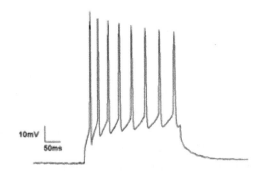

"Current Clamp" is a common technique in electrophysiology. This is a whole cell current clamp recording of a neuron firing a train of action potentials due to it being depolarized by current injection

Structure and Formation of Synapses

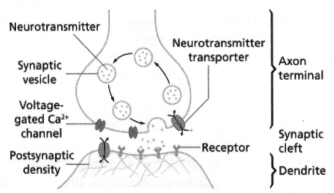

Illustration of the major elements in a prototypical synapse. Synapses are gaps between nerve cells. These cells convert their electrical impulses into bursts of neurochemical relayers, called neurotransmitters, which travel across the synapses to receptors on the dendrites of adjacent cells, thereby triggering further electrical impulses to travel down the latter cells.

Neurons communicate with one another via synapses. Synapses are specialized junctions between two cells in close apposition to one another. In a synapse, the neuron that sends the signal is the presynaptic neuron and the target cell receives that signal is the postsynaptic neuron or cell. Synapses can be either electrical or chemical. Electrical synapses are characterized by the formation of gap junctions that allow ions and other organic compound to instantaneously pass from one cell to another. Chemical synapses are characterized by the presynaptic release of neurotransmitters that diffuse across a synaptic cleft to bind with postsynaptic receptors. A neurotransmitter is a chemical messenger that is synthesized within neurons themselves and released by these same neurons to communicate with their postsynaptic target cells. A receptor is a transmembrane protein molecule that a neurotransmitter or drug binds. Chemical synapses are slower than electrical synapses.

Neurotransmitter Transporters, Receptors, and Signaling Mechanisms

After neurotransmitters are synthesized, they are packaged and stored in vesicles. These vesicles are pooled together in terminal boutons of the presynaptic neuron. When there is a change in voltage in the terminal bouton, voltage-gated calcium channels embedded in the membranes of these boutons become activated. These allow Ca^{2+} ions to diffuse through these channels and bind with synaptic vesicles within the terminal boutons. Once bounded with Ca^{2+}, the vesicles dock and fuse with the presynaptic membrane, and release neurotransmitters into the synaptic cleft by a process known as exocytosis. The neurotransmitters then diffuse across the synaptic cleft and bind to postsynaptic receptors embedded on the postsynaptic membrane of another neuron. There are two families of receptors: ionotropic and metabotropic receptors. Ionotropic receptors are a combination of a receptor and an ion channel. When ionotropic receptors are activated, certain ion species such as Na^+ to enter the postsynaptic neuron, which depolarizes the postsynaptic membrane. If more of the same type of postsynaptic receptors are activated, then more Na^+ will enter the postsynaptic membrane and depolarize cell. Metabotropic receptors on the other hand activate second messenger cascade systems that result in the opening of ion channel located some place else on the same postsynaptic membrane. Although slower than ionotropic receptors that function as on-and-off switches, metabotropic receptors have the advantage of changing the cell's responsiveness to ions and other metabolites, examples being gamma amino-butyric acid (inhibitory transmitter), glutamic acid (excitatory transmitter), dopamine, norepinephrine, epinephrine, melanin, serotonin, melatonin, and substance P.

Postsynaptic depolarizations can be either excitatory or inhibitory. Those that are excitatory are referred to as excitatory postsynaptic potential (EPSP). Alternatively, some postsynaptic receptors allow Cl^- ions to enter the cell or K^+ ions to leave the cell, which results in an inhibitory postsynaptic potential (IPSP). If the EPSP is dominant, the threshold of excitation in the postsynaptic neuron may be reached, resulting in the generation and propagation of an action potential in the postynaptic neuron.

Synaptic Plasticity

Synaptic plasticity is the process whereby strengths of synaptic connections are altered. For example, long-term changes in synaptic connection may result in more postsynaptic receptors being embedded in the postsynaptic membrane, resulting in the strengthening of the synapse. Synaptic plasticity is also found to be the neural mechanism that underlies learning and memory. The basic properties, activity and regulation of membrane currents, synaptic transmission and synaptic plasticity, neurotransmisson, neuroregensis, synaptogenesis and ion channels of cells are a few other fields studied by cellular neuroscientists. Tissue, cellular and subcellular anatomy are studied to provide insight into mental retardation at the Mental Retardation Research Center MRRC Cellular Neuroscience Core. Journals such as *Frontiers in Cellular Neuroscience* and *Molecular and Cellular Neuroscience* are published regarding cellular neuroscientific topics.

Neurophysiology

Neurophysiology is a branch of physiology and neuroscience that is concerned with the study of the functioning of the nervous system. The primary tools of basic neurophysiological research include electrophysiological recordings, such as patch clamp, voltage clamp, extracellular single-unit recording and recording of local field potentials, as well as some of the methods of calcium imaging, optogenetics, and molecular biology.

Neurophysiology is related to electrophysiology, neurobiology, psychology, neurology, clinical neurophysiology, neuroanatomy, cognitive science, biophysics, mathematical biology, and other sciences concerning the brain.

History

Neurophysiology has been a subject of study since as early as 4,000 B.C.

In the early B.C. years, most studies were of different natural sedatives like alcohol and poppy plants. In 1700 B.C., the Edwin Smith surgical papyrus was written. This papyrus was crucial in understanding how the ancient Egyptians understood the nervous system. This papyrus looked at different case studies about injuries to different parts of the body, most notably the head. Beginning around 460 B.C., Hippocrates began to study epilepsy, and theorized that it had its origins in the brain. Hippocrates also theorized that the brain was involved in sensation, and that it was where intelligence was derived from. Hippocrates, as well as most ancient Greeks, believed that relaxation and a stress free environment was crucial in helping treat neurological disorders. In 280 B.C., Erasistratus of Chios theorized that there were divisions in the vestibular processing the brain, as well as deducing from observation that sensation was located there.

In 177 Galen theorized that human thought occurred in the brain, as opposed to the heart as Aristotle had theorized. The optic chiasm, which is crucial to the visual system, was discovered around 100 C.E. by Marinus. Circa 1000, Al-Zahrawi, living in Iberia, began to write about different surgical treatments for neurological disorders. In 1216, the first anatomy textbook in Europe, which included a description of the brain, was written by Mondino de Luzzi. In 1402, St Mary of Bethlehem Hospital (later known as Bedlam in Britain) was the first hospital used exclusively for the mentally ill.

In 1504, Leonardo da Vinci continued his study of the human body with a wax cast of the human ventricle system. In 1536, Nicolo Massa described the effects of different diseases, such as syphilis on the nervous system. He also noticed that the ventricular cavities were filled with cerebrospinal fluid. In 1542, the term physiology was used for the first time by a French physician named Jean Fernel, to explain bodily function in relation to the brain. In 1543, Andreas Vesalius wrote De humani corporis fabrica, which revolutionized the study of anatomy. In this book, he described the pineal gland and what he believed the function was, and was able to draw the corpus striatum which is made up of the basal ganglia and the internal capsule. In 1549, Jason Pratensis (nl) published De Cerebri Morbis. This book was devoted to neurological diseases, and discussed symptoms, as well as ideas from Galen and other Greek, Roman and Arabic authors. It also looked into the anatomy and specific functions of different areas. In 1550, Andreas Vesalius worked on a case of hydrocephalus, or fluid filling the brain. In the same year, Bartolomeo Eustachi studied the optic nerve, mainly focusing on its origin in the brain. In 1564, Giulio Cesare Aranzio discovered the hippocampus, naming it such due to its shape resemblance to a sea horse.

In 1621, Robert Burton published The Anatomy of Melancholy, which looked at the loss of important characters in one's life as leading to depression. In 1649, René Descartes studied the pineal gland. He mistakenly believed that it was the "soul" of the brain, and believed it was where thoughts formed. In 1658, Johann Jakob Wepfer studied a patient in which he believed that a broken blood vessel had caused apoplexy, or a stroke.

In 1749, David Hartley published Observations on Man, which focused on frame (neurology), duty (moral psychology) and expectations (spirituality) and how these integrated within one another. This text was also the first to use the English term psychology. In 1752, the Society of Friends created an asylum in Philadelphia, Pennsylvania. The asylum intended to give not only medical treatment to those mentally ill, but also provide with caretakers and comfortable living conditions. In 1755, Jean-Baptiste Le Roy began using electroconvulsive therapy for the mentally ill, a treatment still used today in specific cases. In 1760, Arne-Charles studied how different lesions in the cerebellum could affect motor movements. In 1776, Vincenzo Malacarne (it) studied the cerebellum intensely, and published a book solely based on its function and appearance.

In 1784, Félix Vicq-d'Azyr, discovered a black colored structure in the midbrain. In 1791 Samuel Thomas von Sömmerring alluded to this structure, calling it the substantia nigra. In the same year, Luigi Galvani described the role of electricity in nerves of dissected frogs. In 1808, Franz Joseph Gall studied and published work on phrenology. Phrenology was the faulty science of looking at head shape to determine different aspects of personality and brain function. In 1811, Julien Jean César Legallois (de) studied respiration in animal dissection and lesions and found the center of respiration in the medulla oblongata. In the same year, Charles Bell finished work on what would later become known as the Bell-Magendie law, which compared functional differences between dorsal and ventral roots of the spinal cord. In 1822, Karl Friedrich Burdach distinguished between the lateral and medial geniculate bodies, as well as named the cingulate gyrus. In 1824, F. Magendie studied and produced the first evidence of the cerebellum's role in equilibration to complete the Bell-Magendie law. In 1838, Theodor Schwann began studying white and grey matter in the brain, and discovered the myelin sheath. These cells, which cover the axons of the neurons in the brain, are named Schwann cells after him. In 1848, Phineas Gage, the classical neurophysiology patient, had his brain pierced by an iron tamping rod in a blasting accident. He became an excellent case study in the connection between the prefrontal cortex and behavior, decision making and consequences. In 1849, Hermann von Helmholtz studied the speed of frog nerve impulses while studying electricity in the body.

While these are certainly not all the developments in neurophysiology before 1849, these developments were significant to the study of the brain and body.

References

- Rutecki, PA. "Neuronal excitability: voltage-dependent currents and synaptic transmission.". Journal of Clinical Neurophysiology. 9: 195–211. doi:10.1097/00004691-199204010-00003. PMID 1375602

- Al, Martini, Frederic Et. Anatomy and Physiology' 2007 Ed.2007 Edition. Rex Bookstore, Inc. p. 288. ISBN 978-971-23-4807-5

- Davies, Melissa (2002-04-09). "The Neuron: size comparison". Neuroscience: A journey through the brain. Retrieved 2009-06-20

- Alvarez-Buylla A, Garcia-Verdugo JM (February 1, 2002). "Neurogenesis in adult subventricular zone". Journal of Neuroscience. 22 (3): 629–34. PMID 11826091. Retrieved 2009-06-20

- Eckert, Roger; Randall, David (1983). Animal physiology: mechanisms and adaptations. San Francisco: W.H. Freeman. p. 239. ISBN 0-7167-1423-X

- Kolodin, YO; Veselovskaia, NN; Veselovsky, NS; Fedulova, SA. Ion conductances related to shaping the repetitive firing in rat retinal ganglion cells. Acta Physiologica Congress. Retrieved 2009-06-20

- Cochilla, AJ; Alford, S (1997). "Glutamate receptor-mediated synaptic excitation in axons of the lamprey". The Journal of Physiology. 499 (Pt 2): 443–57. doi:10.1113/jphysiol.1997.sp021940. PMC 1159318 . PMID 9080373

- Patlak, Joe; Gibbons, Ray (2000-11-01). "Electrical Activity of Nerves". Action Potentials in Nerve Cells. Archived from the original on August 27, 2009. Retrieved 2009-06-20

- Bear, Mark F.; Connors, Barry W.; Paradiso, Michael A. (2006). Neuroscience: Exploring the Brain. Lippincott Williams & Wilkins. p. 13. ISBN 9780781760034

- Sabbatini R.M.E. April–July 2003. Neurons and Synapses: The History of Its Discovery. Brain & Mind Magazine, 17. Retrieved March 19, 2007

- "The Clinical Neurophysiology Primer" By Andrew S. Blum, Seward B. Rutkove, Humana Press, 2007, ISBN 0-89603-996-X, 9780896039964

- Boeing, G. (2016). "Visual Analysis of Nonlinear Dynamical Systems: Chaos, Fractals, Self-Similarity and the Limits of Prediction". Systems. 4 (4): 37. doi:10.3390/systems4040037. Retrieved 2016-12-02

- Swanson, LW. Neuroanatomical terminology : a lexicon of classical origins and historical foundations. Oxford University Press, 2014. England ISBN 9780195340624

- "Cellular Neuroscience" (pdf). Cellular neuroscience research at the University of Victoria. University of Victoria. Retrieved 2008-12-26

Neuron Models in Computational Neuroscience

The section combines neurons' electrophysiological basis of electrical signaling and its anatomy. The components of neural signaling include signal propagation along the dendrite towards the soma, signal propagation along the axon, spatial and temporal summation in the soma, and neurotransmission across the synapse. The text also focuses on concepts of artificial neuron, FitzHugh–Nagumo model, Morris–Lecar model, etc.

Modeling Components of Neuron

The aim of this chapter is to present the modeling components that would constitute a model of a whole neuron.

To begin with let us quickly recall the four components of neural signaling or, rather, the four stages of a neural signal in its passage from the "input" (apical dendrite) of a neuron to its "output" (axon terminal).

1) signal propagation along the dendrite towards the soma

2) spatial and temporal summation in the soma

3) signal propagation along the axon

4) neurotransmission across the synapse

We had also noted earlier that signal propagation along dendrites is mostly passive, as along an electrical cable; that summation occurs in the axon hillock; that an intact action potential propagates down the axon without losing amplitude because it is charged all along the way by voltage-sensitive channels; that neurotransmission occurs across a synapse – as though there is a "hotline" from axon terminal A to apical dendrite B – via chemical means; and, finally, that this whole sequence of events occurs in a neat unidirectional fashion from the apical dendrites to axon terminals.

Dendrite

We introduce three electrical parameters of a dendritic cable. The parameters are defined per unit length of the cable.

1. Axial resistance: Resistance offered by the intracellular compartment per unit length of the cable of diameter, d. The resistivity of the intracellular medium is R_i. We now relate the

resistivity, R_i, which is an intrinsic property of the intracellular medium, to axial resistance, r_a, which is resistance per unit length of the cable.

In general the resistance, R, and resistivity, ρ, of a pipe of area of cross-section, A, and length, L, are related as:

R = ρ L/A, and

Resistance per unit length of the pipe is:

= ρ/A

A similar relation for our cable is:

$$r_a = \frac{R_i}{A} = \frac{R_i}{\pi d^2 / 4} = \frac{4R_i}{\pi d^2} \qquad (\Omega / cm)$$

2. Membrane resistance: The membrane offers resistance for flow current between the intracellular compartment and the extracellular space. This resistance is inversely proportional to the surface area of the membrane.

Therefore, if R_m is the resistance of a membrane patch of unit area, a quantity referred to as specific resistance, the total resistance offered by a cylinder of diameter, d, and unit length, is given as:

$$r_m = \frac{R_m}{A} = \frac{R_m}{\pi d.1} = \frac{R_m}{\pi d} \qquad (\Omega - cm)$$

3. Membrane capacitance: The plasma membrane has a specific capacitance, C_m, of about 10^-6 F/cm^2. Therefore, capacitance of the cable of unit length, c_m, is,

$$c_m = C_m \pi d \qquad (F / cm)$$

Using the electrical parameters defined above, we can now represent the cable as an electric circuit. In this circuit, the continuous cable is represented as a series of discrete circuit elements, in which each element approximates a short length of the cable, say, of length, Δx.

Infinite Cable

Applying Ohm's law to one of the horizontal resistances, r_a Δx,

$$V_m(x,t) - V_m(x + \Delta x, t) = \Delta x r_a I_i(x,t)$$

$$-\frac{\partial V_m}{\partial x} = r_a I_i(x,t)$$

Applying the law of continuity of current at a given node in the circuit of figure,

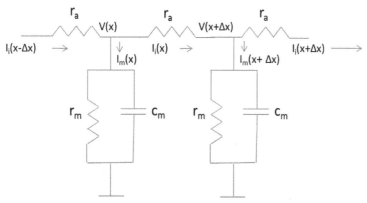

Circuit equivalent for a dendrite

$$I_i(x,t) - I_i(x - \Delta x, t) = -\Delta x I_m(x,t)$$

$$-\frac{\partial I_i}{\partial x} = I_m(x,t)$$

Combining both,

$$\frac{1}{r_a}\frac{\partial^2 V_m}{\partial x^2} = I_m(x,t)$$

Now, the membrane current, I_m, can be resolved into three components 1) current through membrane capacitance, 2) current through membrane resistance, and 3) externally injected current, I_{ext}, if any. Thus,

$$I_m(x,t) = \frac{V_m - V_{rest}}{r_m} + C_m\frac{\partial V_m}{\partial t} - I_{ext}$$

Combining both,

$$\lambda^2\frac{\partial^2 V_m}{\partial x^2} = V_m - V_{rest} + \tau_m\frac{\partial V_m}{\partial t} - r_m I_{ext}$$

where

$\lambda = \sqrt{\dfrac{r_m}{r_a}}$ known as the space constant, and,

$\tau_m = r_m c_m$ known as the time constant, of the cable.

Equation is known as the Linear Cable Equation. Eqn. can be further simplified if the membrane voltage, , is defined with reference to the resting potential. Assuming that the resting potential is the same everywhere along the cable, it only offsets the membrane potential and does not affect the derivative terms in eqn. Thus, from now on, if we designate V_m to represent the deviation of membrane potential from the resting potential, V_{rest}, the (V_m-V_{rest}) term in eqn. can be replaced by, V_m, and we have the following simpler form.

$$\lambda^2\frac{\partial^2 V_m}{\partial x^2} = V_m + \tau_m\frac{\partial V_m}{\partial t} - r_m I_{ext}$$

Steady State Analysis

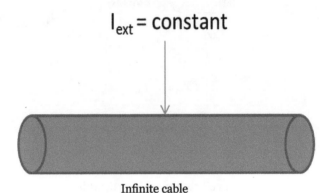

$$I_{ext} = constant$$

Infinite cable

Though our ultimate objective is to be able to describe signal transmission along the cables with complex geometries, we begin with a simple situation.

We consider an infinite cable in which a constant current is injected at a point. The goal is to determine membrane voltage distribution under steady state conditions.

External Current:

$$I_{ext} = I_0\, \delta(x)u(t),$$

spatially it is a point source; and temporally it is a step function.

Boundary conditions:

$$V(x, t) = 0,\ at\ |x| \rightarrow \infty, \forall t$$

Initial condition:

$$V(x, 0) = 0, x \in (-\infty, \infty)$$

Under steady state conditions,

$$\frac{\partial V_m}{\partial t} = 0$$

Therefore, eqn. becomes,

$$\lambda^2 \frac{\partial^2 V_m}{\partial x^2} = V_m - r_m I_{ext}$$

Solution to eqn. will be of the form:

$$V_m(x) = Ae^{x/\lambda} + Be^{-x/\lambda}$$

Since we are concerned with only steady state behavior, time is omitted, and membrane voltage is represented as, $V_m(x)$.

Now let us apply the boundary conditions eqn., to the solution eqn. Since $V_m(x)$ tends to 0 at $+\infty$

, A=0, and since $V_m(x)=0$ at $-\infty$, B = 0. This difficulty can be overcome if we let the form of the solution be

$$V_m(x) = V_o e^{-|x|/l}$$

where V_o is the steady state voltage at x=0.

Let us try to verify that $V_m(x)$ of eqn. satisfies.

$$\frac{\partial V_m(x)}{\partial x} = -\frac{V_0}{\lambda} e^{-|x|/\lambda} sign(x)$$

$$\frac{\partial^2 V_m(x)}{\partial x^2} = -\frac{V_0}{\lambda^2} e^{-|x|/\lambda} - 2\frac{V_0}{\lambda} e^{-|x|/\lambda} \delta(x) = \frac{V_0}{\lambda^2} e^{-|x|/\lambda} - 2\frac{V_0}{\lambda} \delta(x)$$

$$\lambda^2 \frac{\partial^2 V_m(x)}{\partial x^2} = V_0 e^{-|x|/\lambda} - 2V_0 \lambda \delta(x)$$

Comparing the last equation with eqn., we have

$$2\lambda V_o = I_o r_m$$

Or,

$$V_0 = \frac{I_0 r_m}{2\lambda}$$

Therefore, the final form of steady state membrane voltage of an infinite cylinder is,

$$V_m(x) = \frac{I_0 r_m}{2\lambda} e^{-|x|/\lambda}$$

Where

$$\lambda = \sqrt{\frac{r_m}{r_a}} = \sqrt{\frac{R_m}{R_i} \cdot \frac{d}{4}}$$

Electrotonic Distance:

Any length, l, can be expressed as electrotonic distance, L, as,

$$L = \frac{1}{\lambda}$$

Input Resistance

Input resistance, R_{in}, is defined as the ratio of voltage at the point of current injection to the magnitude of current injected.

$$R_{in} = \frac{V(x=0)}{I_0} = \frac{r_m}{2\lambda} = \frac{\sqrt{r_a r_m}}{2}$$

Example:

Consider a infinite cable with the static current $I_0 = 10$ mA injected at point x=2. Plot the static solution for such a cable.

Solution:

The static solution for the infinite cable is given by: $V_m(x) = \dfrac{I_0 r_m}{2\lambda} e^{-|x|/\lambda}$

Since current $I_0 = 10$ mA is injected at x=2, $I_{ext} = I_0 \, \delta(x)$;

The plot of $2V_m(x)/I_0 r_m$ vs x/λ would be:

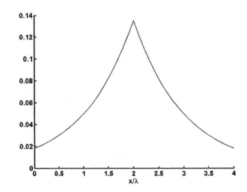

Semi-infinite Cable

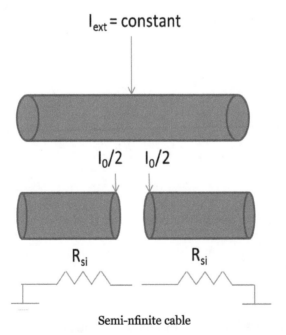

Semi-nfinite cable

Let us consider the case of a semi-infinite cable where current of magnitude, I_0, is injected into one end of the cylinder. Since an infinite cable can be viewed as two semi-infinite cables in parallel, steady state membrane voltage of a semi-infinite cable is twice that of the infinite cable, and is given as,

$$V_m(x) = \frac{I_0 r_m}{\lambda} e^{-|x|/\lambda}$$

Similarly, the input resistance, which is naturally twice that of an infinite cable, is,

$$R_{in} = \frac{V(x=0)}{I_0} = \frac{r_m}{\lambda} = \sqrt{r_a r_m} = r_a \lambda \equiv R_\infty$$

R_∞ is called the input resistance of a semi-infinite cable.

Finite Cable

Consider a finite cable of electrotonic length L. Let X denote the electrotonic distance along the cable,

$$X = \frac{x}{\lambda}$$

A general expression for steady state membrane voltage, as a function of X, is given as,

$$V_m(X) = A \cosh(L - X) + B \sinh(L - X)$$

where,
$$\cosh(x) = (e^x + e^{-x})/2$$

$$\sinh(x) = (e^x - e^{-x})/2$$

Now we consider three different boundary conditions under which we solve the steady state voltage distribution of a finite length cable.

Sealed-end Boundary Condition

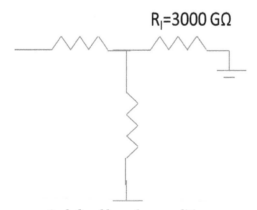

$R_l = 3000\ G\Omega$

Sealed end boundary condition

Physically this refers to the situation when the dendrite is sealed/closed with a membrane patch. Electrically this is equivalent to loading the circuit of figure. at the far end with a resistance equal to that of membrane patch that sealed the dendritic cable. For dendritic cable of diameter, d of 2μm , and R_m of $10^5\ \Omega cm^2$, the loading resistance R_L is,

$$R_L = 3000\ G\Omega$$

$$R_L = \frac{R_m}{\pi d^2 / 4} = 3000 G\Omega$$

Since the sealed end has high resistance we can approximate it with an open circuit, implying that axial current, $I_i = 0$ at the sealed end (X=L).

Therefore, from eqn. ,

$$\left.\frac{\partial V_m}{\partial X}\right|_{X=L} = 0$$

Substituting the above boundary condition in the solution of eqn., we have,

$$\left.\frac{\partial V_m}{\partial X}\right|_{X=L} = -A\sinh(L-X) - B\cosh(L-X) = 0$$

or,

B=0.

Therefore,

$$V_m(X) = A\cosh(L-X)$$

Assuming, V_0, is the voltage at the near-end (x=0=X) of the cable at steady state, the solution can be written as,

$$V_m(X) = V_0 \cosh(L-X) / \cosh(L)$$

$$I_i = -\frac{1}{r_a}\frac{\partial V_m}{\partial x} = \frac{V_0}{\cosh(L)}(-\sinh L - X)(-\frac{1}{r_a \lambda}) = \frac{V_0}{R_\infty}\frac{\sinh(L-X)}{\cosh(L)}$$

At X=0, Ii is,

$$= \frac{V_0}{R_\infty}\tanh(L)$$

$$\therefore R_{in} = R_\infty \coth(L)$$

Killed End Boundary Condition

The previous case of 'sealed-end boundary condition' refers to the situation when the far end is an open circuit. The present case of 'killed end boundary condition' the end of the terminal is 'shorted' so that the voltage at the far end is zero. Physically this situation can be created by cutting ("killing") the far end so that the interior of the dendrite is directly in contact with the extracellular space.

The form of the solution for this case is again,

$$V(X) = A\cosh(L-X) + B\sinh(L-X)$$

Boundary conditions:

$$V(X) = 0 \ at \ X = L$$

$$\therefore A = 0$$

$$V(X) = V_0 \ at \ X = 0$$

$$\therefore B = \frac{V_0}{\sinh(L)}$$

Input resistance: $V(X)/I_i(X)$ at X = 0. Input current is,

$$I_i = -\frac{1}{r_a} \frac{\partial V}{\partial x}\bigg|_{X=0}$$

$$\frac{\partial V}{\partial X} = -V_0 \frac{\cosh(L-X)}{\sinh(L)}$$

$$\therefore I_i = -\frac{1}{r_a} \frac{\partial V}{\partial x}\bigg|_{x=0} = \frac{V_0}{r_a} \coth(L)$$

$$\therefore R_{in} = \frac{V_0}{I_i} = \lambda r_a \tanh(L) = R_\infty \tanh(L)$$

Arbitrary Boundary Condition

Let load resistance be = R_L. Load voltage = V_L.

$$V(X) = A\cosh(L-X) + B\sinh(L-X)$$

Boundary conditions:

$$V(X) = V_L \ at \ X = L$$

$$\therefore A = V_L$$

$$V(X) = V_0 \ at \ X = 0$$

$$\therefore B = \frac{V_0 - V_L \cosh(L)}{\sinh(L)}$$

Substituting...

$$V(X) = V_L \cosh(L-X) + \frac{(V_0 - V_L \cosh(L))}{\sinh(L)} \sinh(L-X)$$

$$= \frac{V_L \cosh(L-X)\sinh(L) + (V_0 - V_L \cosh(L))\sinh(L-X)}{\sinh(L)}$$

$$\frac{V_L \cosh(L-X)\sinh(L) + V_0 \sinh(L-X) - V_L \cosh(L)\sinh(L-X)}{\sinh(L)}$$

(Using, $\sinh(X) = \sinh(L - (L-X)) = \sinh(L)\cosh(L-X) - \sinh(L-X)\cosh(L))$

$$= \frac{V_L \sinh(X) + V_0 \sinh(L - X)}{\sinh(L)}$$

$$= \frac{V_L \cosh(L - X)\sinh(L) + V_0 \sinh(L - X) - V_L \cosh(L)\sinh(L - X)}{\sinh(L)}$$

(Using, $\sinh(X) = \sinh(L - (L-X)) = \sinh(L)\cosh(L-X) - \sinh(L-X)\cosh(L))$

$$= \frac{V_L \sinh(X) + V_0 \sinh(L - X)}{\sinh(L)}$$

Axial current is,

$$I_i(X) = -\frac{1}{r_a}\frac{\partial V}{\partial X} = -\frac{1}{r_a\lambda}\frac{V_L \cosh(X) - V_0 \cosh(L - X)}{\sinh(L)}$$

Current flowing into the load is, $I_i(X)$ at $X = L$, which is,

$$I_i = -\frac{1}{r_a}\frac{\partial V}{\partial X} = -\frac{1}{r_a\lambda}\frac{V_L \cosh(L) - V_0}{\sinh(L)}$$

Since load current is also equal to, V_L / R_L, we have

$$-\frac{1}{r_a\lambda}\frac{V_L \cosh(L) - V_0}{\sinh(L)} = \frac{V_L}{R_L},$$

or,

$$V_L = \frac{V_0 R_L}{R_\infty \sinh(L) + R_L \cosh(L)}$$

$$= \frac{V_0}{\dfrac{R_\infty}{R_L}\sinh(L) + \cosh(L)}$$

Substituting the above in eqn.,

$$V(X) = \frac{V_L \sinh(X) + V_0 \sinh(L - X)}{\sinh(L)}$$

$$= \frac{V_0 \sinh(L-X) + \dfrac{V_0}{\dfrac{R_\infty}{R_L}\sinh(L)+\cosh(L)} \sinh(X)}{\sinh(L)}$$

$$= V_0 \frac{(\dfrac{R_\infty}{R_L}\sinh(L)+\cosh(L))\sinh(L-X)+\sinh(X)}{\sinh(L)(\dfrac{R_\infty}{R_L}\sinh(L)+\cosh(L))}$$

$$= V_0 \frac{\dfrac{R_\infty}{R_L}\sinh(L)\sinh(L-X)+\cosh(L)\sinh(L-X)+\sinh(L-(L-X))}{\sinh(L)(\dfrac{R_\infty}{R_L}\sinh(L)+\cosh(L))}$$

$$= V_0 \frac{\dfrac{R_\infty}{R_L}\sinh(L)\sinh(L-X)+\sinh(L)\cosh(L-X)}{\sinh(L)(\dfrac{R_\infty}{R_L}\sinh(L)+\cosh(L))}$$

On further reduction we obtain,

$$V(X) = V_0 \frac{\dfrac{R_\infty}{R_L}\sinh(L-X)+\cosh(L-X)}{(\dfrac{R_\infty}{R_L}\sinh(L)+\cosh(L))}$$

Applying the formula for the input current,

$$I_i = -\frac{1}{r_a}\frac{\partial V}{\partial x}\Big|_{x=0}$$

We can obtain the expression for Rin as,

$$R_{in} = \frac{V_0}{I_i(X=0)} = R_\infty \frac{R_\infty \tanh(L)+R_L}{R_L \tanh(L)+R_\infty}$$

Time-dependent Solution

$$\lambda^2 \frac{\partial^2 V_m}{\partial x^2} = \tau \frac{\partial V_m}{\partial t} + V_m - I_{inj}r_m$$

Let,

$$T = \frac{t}{\tau_m}; \quad X = \frac{x}{\lambda}$$

$$\frac{\partial^2 V_m}{\partial x^2} = \frac{\partial V_m}{\partial t} + V_m - \frac{I_{inj}(X,T)}{\lambda c_m}$$

$$I_{inj}(X,T) = \lambda \tau_m I_{inj}(x,t) \quad (current\ density)$$

Infinite Cable

Impulse Response

Boundary condition: $V(X) \rightarrow 0,\ as\ |X| \rightarrow \infty$

$$If, I_{inj} = I_0 = \frac{Q_0}{\tau_m} \quad (an\ infintely\ breif\ pulse)$$

$$V(X,T) = \frac{I_0 r_m}{2\lambda\sqrt{\pi T}} e^{-\frac{X^2}{4T}} . e^{-T}$$

For long times, decay pattern is the same throughout the cable.

Since the system is linear, response to arbitrary current injection is given as,

$$V(X,T) = \frac{\tau_m}{Q_0} V_\delta(X,T) * I_{inj}(T)$$

$$= \frac{\tau_m}{Q_0} \int V_\delta(X,T') * I_{inj}(T-T') dT'$$

Voltage response to current step:

$$I_{inj} = I_{step} = I_o u(t)$$

$$V(X,T) = I_o \frac{\tau_m}{Q_0} \int_0^T V_\delta(X,T') dt'$$

$$V_{step}(0,T) = \frac{I_0 R_\infty}{2} erf(\sqrt{T})$$

Example:

Plot the time dependant solutions for different distances from the point of injection for a semi- infinite cable with respect to time. Current is injected at X=0;

Solution:

The required plots can be generated using the formula:

$$V(X,T) = \frac{I_0 R_m}{\lambda \sqrt{\pi T}} e^{-\frac{X^2}{4T}} e^{-T}$$

Approximating it as:

$$V(X,T) = B.e^{-\frac{X^2}{4T}} e^{-T}$$

We plot the X's(distance's) at intervals of 0.5.

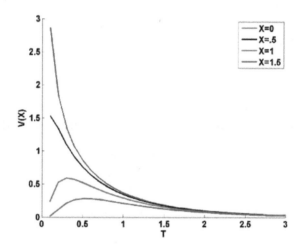

Propagation Delay

Linear cable equation does not admit any wave equation, due to dissipation of energy through the passive membrane. If voltage-sensitive, nonlinear elements are sensitive, then we can have traveling waves as it happens in the axons.

One way of defining velocity is by tracking motion of the peak. But a centroid gives uniform propagation velocity.

$$\hat{t}_x^h = \frac{\int\limits_{-\infty}^{\infty} th(x,t)dt}{\int\limits_{-\infty}^{\infty} h(x,t)dt}$$

Transfer Delay

Transfer delay is the difference in centroid of induced voltage at y, and the centroid of injected current at 'x'.

$$D_{x \to y} = D_{xy} = \hat{t}_x^V - \hat{t}_x^I$$

Input or local delay:

$$D_{xx} = \hat{t}_x^V - \hat{t}_x^I$$

- D_{xy} is always positive and is independent of the shape of the transient input current.
- It is the property of the cable and not of the input waveform

No matter what the electrical structure of the cable, the transfer delay is symmetric.

$$D_{xy} = D_{yx}$$

It does not depend on the direction of travel. Isopotential neuron – membrane patch:

$$D_{xx} = \tau_m$$

Infinite or semi-infinite cable:

$$D_{xx} = \frac{\tau_m}{2}$$

If the current is injected at x and the voltage is recorded at y, the two centroids are displaced by,

$$D_{xx} = (1 + \frac{|x - y|}{\lambda}) \frac{\tau_m}{2}$$

Propagation delay in difference between centroids of voltage at x and y:

$$P_{xy} = \hat{t}_y^V - \hat{t}_x^V = D_{xy} - D_{xx}$$

For an infinite cable,

$$P_{xx} = (\frac{|x - y|}{\lambda}) \frac{\tau_m}{2}$$

$$v = \frac{distance}{delay} = \frac{2\lambda}{\tau_m} = (\frac{d}{R_m R_i C_m^2})^{1/2} \quad "pseudo - velocity"$$

Branched Cables

Assume that the 2 rightmost branches terminate with sealed end (open) boundary conditions. Input resistance of the branches,

$$R_{in,1} = R_{\infty,1} coth(L_1)$$

$$R_{in,2} = R_{\infty,2} coth(L_2)$$

Terminal resistance of main cable, $R_{L,0}$ is given as,

$$\frac{1}{R_{L,0}} = \frac{1}{R_{in,1}} + \frac{1}{R_{in,2}}$$

Given the terminal resistance, the input resistance is calculated as,

$$R_{in,o} = R_{\infty,0} \frac{R_{L,0} + R_{\infty,0} \tanh(L_0)}{R_{\infty,0} + R_{L,0} \tanh(L_0)}$$

Moving from outermost dendritic tips, one moves towards the soma. Finally at X=0, in the parent cable,

$$V_0 = R_{in,0} I_{inj}$$

Given V0, we can use, voltage distribution along the main branch is,

$$V(X) = V_0 \frac{\frac{R_\infty}{R_L} \sinh(L-X) + \cosh(L-X)}{(\frac{R_\infty}{R_L} \sinh(L) + \cosh(L))}$$

From the above, we can calculate V12, the voltage at the bifurcation point as,

$$V_{12} = V(x)|_{X=L} \frac{V_0}{(\frac{R_\infty}{R_L} \sinh(L) + \cosh(L))}$$

Voltage distribution along the two terminal branches is,

$$V_1(X) = V_{12} \frac{\cosh(L_1 - X)}{\cosh(L_1)}$$

$$V_2(X) = V_{12} \frac{\cosh(L_2 - X)}{\cosh(L_2)}$$

Upward pass (terminals to the root) – compute R_{in}'s::

Compute $R_{in,1}$ and $R_{n,2}$ using eqns. Using $R_{in,1}$ and $R_{n,2}$ compute $R_{L,0}$ using, Eqn. Using all the 3 results compute, $R_{in,0}$ using eqn.

Downward pass (Root to terminals – compute V(x)):

Rall's condition

When the diameters of the two terminal branches are related to the diameter of the main branch in a special way.

$$d_0^{3/2} = d_1^{3/2} + d_2^{3/2}$$

Lengths of the two terminal branches must be the same i.e., $L_1 = L_2 = L$ (say).

$$R_\infty = (R_m R_i)^{1/2} \frac{2}{\pi d^{3/2}} = \frac{a}{d^{3/2}}$$

Therefore,

$$R_{\infty,0} = \frac{a}{d_0^{3/2}}, R_{\infty,1} = \frac{a}{d_1^{3/2}}, R_{\infty,2} = \frac{a}{d_2^{3/2}}$$

Note that, thanks to the way the diameters of the 3 cables are related, we have a special relation among the R_∞'s also,

$$\frac{1}{R_{\infty,0}} = \frac{1}{R_{\infty,1}} + \frac{1}{R_{\infty,2}}$$

Input resistance of the terminal branches are,

$$R_{in,1} = R_{\infty,1} \coth(L) \, and \, R_{in,2} = R_{\infty,2} \coth(L)$$

Thus, terminal resistance of the main cable is given as,

$$\frac{1}{R_{L,0}} = \frac{1}{R_{in,1}} + \frac{1}{R_{in,2}}$$

$$= (\frac{1}{R_{\infty,1}} + \frac{1}{R_{\infty,2}}) \tanh(L)$$

$$= \frac{1}{R_{\infty,0}} \tanh(L)$$

Or,

$$R_{L,0} = R_{\infty,0} \coth(L)$$

From, eqn. we may write down the voltage distribution of the main cable as,

$$V(X) = V_0 \frac{R_{\infty,0} \sinh(L_0 - X) + R_{L,0} \cosh(L_0 - X)}{(R_{\infty,0} \sinh(L_0) + R_{L,0} \cosh(L_0))}$$

Inserting the expression for $R_{L,0}$ from eqn. here,

$$V(X) = V_0 \frac{R_{\infty,0} \sinh(L_0 - X) + R_{\infty,0} \coth(L) \cosh(L_0 - X)}{(R_{\infty,0} \sinh(L_0) + R_{\infty,0} \coth(L) \cosh(L_0))}$$

$$= V_0 \frac{\sinh(L) \sinh(L_0 - X) + \cosh(L) \cosh(L_0 - X)}{\sinh(L) \sinh(L_0) + \cosh(L) \cosh(L_0)}$$

$$= V_0 \frac{\cosh(L_0 + L - X)}{\cosh(L_0 + L)}$$

Rall's Conditions

1) R_m, R_i are the same in all branches

2) All terminals end in the same boundary condition

3) All terminal branches end at the same electrotonic distance from the origin of the main branch

4) At every branch point, infinite input resistances must be matched, i.e.,

$$d_0^{3/2} = \sum_i d_i^{3/2}$$

Where, di are the diameters of the branch cables and do is the diameter of the root cable at the branch cable.

5) Identical synaptic inputs must be delivered to all corresponding dendritic locations.

$$X = L_0 + X_1$$

Axon

From the Hodgkin-Huxley model, we know the mechanisms underlying membrane excitation. We know how currents that exceed a threshold value can produce action potentials. But the Hodgkin-Huxley model is an isopotential model. It applies to a patch of membrane with homogenous distribution of ion channels and a uniform membrane voltage.

Therefore, it does not describe signal propagation. With a slight modification, the Hodgkin-Huxley model can be transformed into a model of voltage wave propagation in an axon.

Eqn. depicts the relationship between the membrane current, I_m, and second spatial derivative of membrane voltage.

$$\frac{1}{r_a} \frac{\partial^2 V_m}{\partial x^2} = I_m(x,t)$$

This relationship can use used to develop a model of action potential propagation in the axon.

Reproducing eqn. here with a slight rearrangement of terms,

$$C\frac{dV_m}{dt} + g_{Na}^{max} m^3 h(V_m - E_{Na}) + g_k^{max} n^4 (V_m - E_K) + g_1(V_m - E_1) = I_{ext}$$

I_{ext} in the above equation represents I_m in eqn. expressed per unit length.

Currents in eqn. are expressed as per unit area, whereas current in eqn. is expressed in per unit length. To describe propagation along a cable, we need to express all membrane currents as per unit length.

From eqn. we know that,

$$r_a = \frac{R_i}{A} = \frac{R_i}{\pi d^2 / 4} = \frac{4R_i}{\pi d^2}$$

For a cable of diameter, d, the membrane current per unit length of the axon is expressed by dividing the currents in eqn. by π*d*1,

$$\frac{1}{\pi d r_a} \frac{\partial^2 V_m}{\partial x^2} = \frac{I_m(x,t)}{\pi d}$$

Or

$$\frac{d}{4R_i} \frac{\partial^2 V_m}{\partial x^2} = \frac{I_m(x,t)}{\pi d}$$

Substituting the last equation in eqn.,

$$\frac{d}{4R_i} \frac{\partial^2 V_m}{\partial x^2} = C \frac{dV_m}{dt} + g_{Na}^{max} m^3 h(V_m - E_{Na}) + g_k^{max} n^4 (V_m - E_K) + g_l(V_m - E_l)$$

Eqn. along with eqns. constitute the complete set of equations that describe signal propagation along an axon.

Eqn. can be written as,

$$\frac{\partial^2 V_m}{\partial x^2} = \frac{4R_i}{d} (C \frac{dV_m}{dt} + g_{Na}^{max} m^3 h(V_m - E_{Na}) + g_k^{max} n^4 (V_m - E_K) + g_l(V_m - E_l))$$

We need to seek propagating wave solutions for the above equation. Assuming the existence of a voltage wave, V(x – u$_t$), propagating with a uniform velocity, u, along the axon, the wave must also satisfy the wave equation,

$$\frac{\partial^2 V_m}{\partial x^2} = \frac{1}{u^2} \frac{\partial^2 V_m}{\partial t^2}$$

Substitution, we may write eqn. as,

$$\frac{1}{K} \frac{\partial^2 V_m}{\partial x^2} = \frac{dV_m}{dt} + \frac{I_{ionic}}{C_m}$$

Where I_{ionic} is the sum of all the ionic currents in eqn. and,

$$K = \frac{4R_i u^2 C_m}{d}$$

Note that the currents are expressed in terms of per unit area, therefore they are independent of the axon diameter, d. Similarly the voltage V_m must also be independent of d. Therefore K must also be independent of d. Since R_i and C_m are independent of d by definition, it implies that u^2/d is independent of d. In other words,

$$u \propto \sqrt{d}$$

Thus we have a relationship between cable diameter and conduction velocity. This rule is roughly followed in real, unmyelinated axons.

Note that the result of eqn. is identical to that of eqn., the derivation is quite different in the two cases.

Just as the Hodgkin-Huxley model, which is an isopotential model, exhibits threshold effect, the model of wave propagation also exhibits a threshold effect. When suprathreshold external current is injected in at a point in an axon, Na$^+$ ions rush in thereby increasing local membrane voltage rapidly. Voltage increase in neighboring regions activate the local Na$^+$ channels further amplifying the voltage buildup. The fraction of membrane current that depolarizes neighboring membrane segments is called 'local circuit current.' As this process continues, the action potential spreads along the axon. When a subthreshold current is injected, the local Na$^+$ channels are not activated, and therefore, due to inadequate amplification, there is no local spread of action potential.

When the current is close to the threshold (within 1% of threshold current), there may not be a propagating wave, but a decaying wave that dies down to resting potential with increasing distance from the point of injection.

Another feature that controls action potential propagation consists of the values of channel conductances. Since the action potential generation and propagation is dependent crucially on voltage-sensitive Na$^+$ and K$^+$ channels, the conductances of these two channels must be sufficiently high for signal propagation. In a simulation study of signal propagation in axon, Cooley and Dodge (1966) reduced gNa and gK by a scaling factor η. They found that for $\eta <= 0.26$, action potential was generated but did no propagate as a stable wave. Only a decaying wave was observed.

Voltage-sensitive Ion Channels

We have seen how we can express channel models in terms of gating variables. Specifically we considered voltage-sensitive Na$^+$ and K$^+$ channels used in the Hodgkin-Huxley model. Both of these models had a common mathematical structure. Channel current, I_x, is expressed as a function of gating variables, an activation variable, m, and an inactivation variable, h, as follows:

$$I_x = \bar{g}m^p h^q (V_m - E_x)$$

In the HH model, p=3 and q = 1 for the Na+ channel, and p=4, q=0 (for the activation variable)

for K$^+$ channel. Separate α and β functions were associated with each channel. The form of the conductance variation is given in eqn., and the α and β functions determine the dynamics of the channel.

We now present models of a greater variety of channels. While the above modeling structure applies to most cases, there will be some deviations. Broadly 4 classes of channels will be considered:

1. Sodium channels

2. Potassium Channels

3. Chloride Channels

4. Calcium channels

   a. Calcium gated potassium channels

Sodium Channels

Sodium channels are broadly classified into "transient" and "persistent" type.

The sodium channels of HH model are fast channels in which the conductance rises fast, due to fast activation dynamics, and drops rapidly, due to fast inactivation dynamics. Such currents are usually called "transient" since the channel opens briefly and shuts again, even though the membrane is depolarized. A transient sodium current, like the one in HH model, can be expressed as,

$$I_{Na,t} = \bar{g}m^3 h(V_m - E_{Na})$$

But there are sodium channels which do not have inactivation gates ie., h variable is absent. Such channels open on depolarization and remain open as long as the membrane remains depolarized. Such sodium channels are said to be "persistent" ($I_{Na,p}$) or "noninactivating" (referring to the absence of inactivation dynamics). $I_{Na,p}$ currents are found for example in the thalamocortical neurons in rats (Parri and Crunelli 1999). A persistent sodium current may be expressed as,

$$I_{Na,p} = \bar{g}m(V_m - E_{Na})$$

Potassium Channels

Voltage-sensitive potassium channels are broadly classified in terms of 1) the speed of their inactivation dynamics, and 2) the direction of the currents. Potassium currents with slow inactivation dynamics are said to be "delayed" while those with fast inactivation dynamics are said to carry "A type" currents.

Channels that allow currents in only one direction are said to be rectifying. "Outward rectifying" channels are those that allow current in the outward direction, while "inward rectifying" channels are that allow currents in inward direction. Thus there are three important classes of voltage-sensitive potassium currents:

1) Delayed rectifier currents: These currents have slow inactivation dynamics and allow currents in the outward direction. (The 'rectifier' implicitly means outward rectifying). The potassium currents in HH model are of this type.

2) A currents: These currents have fast inactivation dynamics.

3) Inward rectifying currents: Those most potassium channels are outward rectifying, there are a special class of potassium channels (sometimes referred to as the "exceptional") that are inward rectifying. These are denoted by K_{IR} channels. These channels open under conditions of hyperpolarization.

Calcium Currents

Like the voltage-sensitive sodium and potassium currents visited above, calcium currents are also described in terms of activation, m, and inactivation, h, variables. But the calcium current cannot be calculated using the simple expression of eqn. since the calcium concentration inside the neuron is very low (O(nM)) and varies rapidly due to calcium flux. Therefore, the Nernst potential formula which depends on assumptions of equilibrium conditions is not valid. The correct formula for calcium current is given as,

$$I_{Ca} = \bar{p}m^p h^q \frac{V_m z^2 F^2}{RT} \frac{\left[Ca^{2+}\right]_e e^{-V_m zF/RT} - \left[Ca^{2+}\right]_i}{1 - e^{-V_m zF/RT}}$$

Where,

$\left[Ca^{2+}\right]_e$ - extracellular calcium concentration (usually about 2 mM).

$\left[Ca^{2+}\right]_i$ - intracellular calcium concentration (varies but low)

$\bar{p}$ - max. permeability to calcium

Faraday's constant, F = 9.648 X 10^4 C mol^{-1}

Ideal gas constant, R = 8.314 V C K^{-1} mol^{-1}

Though the above description is valid for general calcium currents, there are two subcategories of calcium currents which depend on the threshold voltage at which the channels get activated. These are:

1) Low-threshold calcium current (I_T):

   The low threshold calcium channels open at a threshold voltage of about -40 mV. That is, these channels open under conditions of hyperpolarization. Hence IT current is responsible for an interesting phenomenon called *post-inhibitory rebound*. When an inhibitory, hyperpolarizing input is suddenly switched off, a neuron can show a rebound response whereby, the cell might fire a few action potentials, a phenomenon called post-inhibitory rebound. The role of low threshold calcium channels in post- inhibitory rebound may be explained as follows.

   For the low threshold calcium channels under conditions of hyperpolarization (created by inhibitory input), the inactivation variable, h, is positive. But the channel is in closed state since the activation variable, m, is 0. But when the hyperpolarizing current is stopped, membrane voltage gradually increases. Therefore, m gradually increases while h decreases. There will be a critical stage at which both m and h are sufficiently positive, when the channels are briefly open, allowing a transient calcium pulse. Such pulses are known as low-threshold calcium spikes. The resulting calcium influx transiently increase membrane voltage which in turn triggers a couple of sodium spikes.

2) High-threshold calcium current (I_L):

   The IL current differs from its low-threshold counterpart only in the threshold voltage at which the channel gets activated. The High-threshold calcium channels, as the name indicates, open only at high levels of membrane depolarization. They are activated even during the action potentials and contribute to changes in membrane voltage. In addition this class of calcium channels have a role in controlling a class of potassium channels.

2a) Calcium-controlled potassium channels:

Intracellular calcium ions are important players in many forms of second-messenger signaling. An instance of such signaling is the role of intracellular calcium in dynamics of a special class of potassium channels, the calcium-controlled potassium channels. Current through these channels is given as,

$$I_c = \bar{g}_C m (V_m - E_K)$$

Dynamics of the activation variable, m, is given in the usual form, as:

$$\dot{m} = \alpha m - \beta (1-m)$$

In the channels of HH model, the α and β functions only depend on membrane voltage, Vm. But in the present case, α depends on intracellular calcium, $\left[Ca^{2+} \right]_i$ as follows:

$$\alpha = A \left[Ca^{2+} \right]_i \exp(V_m / k)$$

$$\beta = B \left[Ca^{2+} \right]_i \exp(-V_m / k)$$

where A, B and k are constants. We know that steady-state value of m may be expressed in terms of α and β functions as,

$$m_\infty = \alpha / (\alpha + \beta)$$

Thus increasing $\left[Ca^{2+} \right]_i$ can be seen to increase m, and therefore I_C (up to a point of saturation).

Synapse

We have already seen that synaptic transmission converts a presynaptic electrical event viz., action potential, into a postsynaptic electrical event – the PSP. This change is produced by the action of the neurotransmitter on a postsynaptic receptor which leads to opening of an ion channel on the postsynaptic side. Therefore the simplest form modeling a synapse would be to consider a membrane model of the postsynaptic side and describe the transient change in the conductance of the ion channel involved in the transmission event.

Circuit Model of Synapse

Accordingly consider a simple circuit model of the postsynaptic membrane in the figure below.

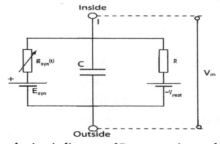

Simple circuit diagram of Post synaptic membrane

$g_{syn}(t)$ – is the time-varying synaptic conductance (of the ion channel involved in synaptic transmission)

E_{syn} – is the Nernst potential corresponding to the ion channel (involved in synaptic transmission) and the ionic species to which it is permeable

C – membrane capacitance

Vrest – resting membrane potential of the postsynaptic membrane

R – membrane resistance

The central and right branches consisting of C, R and V_{rest} together model the passive membrane properties in the absence of synaptic transmission. The left branch becomes active only when there is synaptic transmission, i.e., when $g_{syn}(t) > 0$.

Applying Kirchoff's current law to the above circuit, we have,

$$C\frac{dV_m}{dt} + g_{syn}(t)(V_m - E_{syn}) + \frac{(V_m - V_{rest})}{R} = 0$$

Note that normal resting conditions of the postsynaptic membrane occur by setting $g_{syn}(t) = 0$ and $V_m = V_{rest}$ in the above equation.

The transient increase and return to zero of synaptic conductance $g_{syn}(t)$ is usually expressed in the following form,

$$g_{syn}(t) = Ate^{-t/t_{peak}}$$

Where A is a constant, and t_{peak} is the time at which $g_{syn}(t)$ peaks. Note that the above expression represents variation of synaptic conductance in response to a single action potential.

Since Post Synaptic Potential (PSP) is defined as the deviation from the resting potential, we define a new voltage variable, v, as,

$$v = V_m - V_{rest}$$

Accordingly eqn. may be rewritten as,

$$C\frac{dv}{dt} + g_{syn}(t)(v + V_{rest} - E_{syn}) + \frac{v}{R} = 0$$

Or,

$$C\frac{dv}{dt} = -(g_{syn}(t) + \frac{1}{R})v + g_{syn}(t)(E_{syn} - V_{rest})$$

Therefore, during the neurotransmission, when $g_{syn}(t)$ begins to rise, the sign of $(E_{syn} - V_{rest})$ determines the direction of change in v. We have three cases in order.

Case 1: $E_{syn} > V_{rest}$

This amounts to having a positive injected current n eqn. Therefore v transiently increases. This corresponds to an Excitatory Post Synaptic Potential (EPSP). A common example of synapses that produce such EPSPs is the fast, excitatory synapses with AMPA receptors (or non-NMDA type) and glutamate as neurotransmitter.

Case 2: $E_{syn} < V_{rest}$

Since the current injected is negative, we have a negative deviation in v, which is an Inhibitory Post Synaptic Potential (IPSP).

A common example is the inhibitory synapse with GABA as the neurotransmitter and $GABA_B$ as the receptor. The channel involved is a potassium channel with E_{syn} that is 10-30 mV below the resting potential.

Case 3: $E_{syn} \approx V_{rest}$

There is no current in the synaptic conductance in this case. So it does not seem to have any apparent effect on the postsynaptic potential.

An example of such a synapse is the GABA synapse with GABA_A receptor and chloride as the associated channels. The reversal potential of these channels is close to the resting potential of many cells in which these synapses are found.

Although these synapses do not seem to have any effect in isolation, when used in conjunction with excitatory synapses they show an interesting effect. Let us rewrite eqn, so as to include a synapse in which $E_{syn} \approx V_{rest}$, and an excitatory synapse.

$$C\frac{dv}{dt} = -(g_{syn}^0(t) + g_{syn}^e(t) + \frac{1}{R})v + g_{syn}^0(t)(E_{syn}^0 - V_{rest}) + g_{syn}^e(t)(E_{syn}^e - V_{rest})$$

(g_{syn}^0, E_{syn}^0) - conductance and reversal potential of the synapse where $E_{syn}^0 \approx V_{rest}$

(g_{syn}^e, E_{syn}^e) - conductance and reversal potential of the excitatory synapse

The second term on the RHS is small since $E_{syn}^0 \approx V_{rest}$. But due to the presence of g_{syn}^0 , the conductance term in the first term on RHS is greater (than what it would be when only the excitatory synapse is present). Therefore, under these conditions the EPSP produced is smaller than what it would be when the excitatory synapse alone is present. In that sense, the synapse corresponding to (g_{syn}^0, E_{syn}^0) is inhibiting the excitatory synapse. Therefore it is known as a silent or a shunting inhibition.

Excitatory Synapses

AMPA type synapses: The form of conductance variation of eqn. is applicable for a general synapse. More accurate models have been proposed for specific synapses. A model of synaptic conductance with a double exponential term has been proposed for AMPA synapses (Gabbiani et al 1994):

$$g_{ampa}(t) = \overline{g}_{ampa} A(e^{-t/\tau_{decay}} - e^{-t/\tau_{rise}})H(t)$$

$\overline{g}_{ampa}$: maximum value of the synaptic conductance

A : normalizing constant that ensures that the highest value of the bracketed expression is unity

t_decay, t_rise : decay and rise time constants

H(t): the step function or the Heaviside function

Numerical values of the above parameters used in (Gabbiani 1994) are as follows:

$$\overline{g}_{ampa} = 750\,pS; A = 1.273; t\_decay = 1.5\,ms, t\_rise = 0.09\,ms.$$

NMDA type synapses: This type of synapses have more complex dynamics than AMPA type synapses, since they are dual-gated: they can be gated by both the neurotransmitter and the membrane voltage. Modeling the conductance change due to the neurotransmitter is similar to the cases seen above. Under conditions of normal membrane polarity, extracellular Mg2+ blocks the NMDA associated channels. This block is removed when the membrane potential is depolarized beyond -50 mV. However the time-scales of opening of this channel is longer (10-100 ms) compared to that of AMPA channels (about 1 ms). The form of synaptic conductance for NMDA type synapses is given as follows (Gabbiani et al 1994):

$$g_{nmda}(t) = \overline{g}_{nmda} A(e^{-t/\tau_{decay}} - e^{-t/\tau_{rise}})(1 + e^{\alpha V_m}\left[Mg^{2+}\right]_0 / \beta)H(t)$$

Values of various parameters in the last equation are given as (Gabbiani et al 1994),

$$\overline{g}_{nmda} = 1.2\,nS; A = 1.358; t_{decay} = 40\,ms, t_{rise} = 3\,ms; \alpha = 0.062\,mV^{-1}; \beta = 3.57\,mM;$$

$$\left[Mg^{2+}\right]_0 = 1.2\,mM.$$

Inhibitory Synapses

Even for inhibitory synapses, there are more complex models of synaptic conductance variation than that given by eqn. For example, in the GABAergic synapses of cerebellar granule cells, post-synaptic current is found to have a fast and a slow component. Synaptic conductance in such a case may be expressed as,

$$g_{gaba}(t) = \overline{g}_{gaba}(\overline{g}_{fast}e^{-t/\tau_{fast}} + \overline{g}_{slow}e^{-t/\tau_{slow}})H(t)$$

Artificial Neuron

An artificial neuron is a mathematical function conceived as a model of biological neurons. Artificial neurons are the constitutive units in an artificial neural network. Depending on the specific model used they may be called a semi-linear unit, Nv neuron, binary neuron, linear threshold function, or McCulloch–Pitts (MCP) neuron. The artificial neuron receives one or more inputs (representing dendrites) and sums them to produce an output (or activation) (representing a neuron's axon). Usually the sums of each node are weighted, and the sum is passed through a non-linear function known as an activation function or transfer function. The transfer functions usually have a sigmoid shape, but they may also take the form of other non-linear functions, piecewise linear functions, or step functions. They are also often monotonically increasing, continuous, differentiable and bounded. The thresholding function is inspired to build logic gates referred to as threshold logic; with a renewed interest to build logic circuit resembling brain processing. For example, new devices such as memristors have been extensively used to develop such logic in the recent times.

The artificial neuron transfer function should not be confused with a linear system's transfer function.

Basic Structure

For a given artificial neuron, let there be $m + 1$ inputs with signals x_0 through x_m and weights w_0 through w_m. Usually, the x_0 input is assigned the value +1, which makes it a *bias* input with $w_{k0} = b_k$. This leaves only m actual inputs to the neuron: from x_1 to x_m.

The output of the kth neuron is:

$$y_k = \varphi\left(\sum_{j=0}^{m} w_{kj} x_j\right)$$

Where φ (phi) is the transfer function.

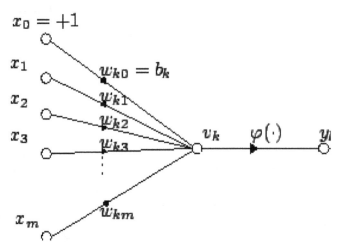

The output is analogous to the axon of a biological neuron, and its value propagates to the input of the next layer, through a synapse. It may also exit the system, possibly as part of an output vector.

It has no learning process as such. Its transfer function weights are calculated and threshold value are predetermined.

Comparison to Biological Neurons

Artificial neurons are designed to mimic aspects of their biological counterparts.

- *Dendrites* – In a biological neuron, the dendrites act as the input vector. These dendrites allow the cell to receive signals from a large (>1000) number of neighboring neurons. As in the above mathematical treatment, each dendrite is able to perform "multiplication" by that dendrite's "weight value." The multiplication is accomplished by increasing or decreasing the ratio of synaptic neurotransmitters to signal chemicals introduced into the dendrite in response to the synaptic neurotransmitter. A negative multiplication effect can be achieved by transmitting signal inhibitors (i.e. oppositely charged ions) along the dendrite in response to the reception of synaptic neurotransmitters.

- *Soma* – In a biological neuron, the soma acts as the summation function, seen in the above mathematical description. As positive and negative signals (exciting and inhibiting, respectively) arrive in the soma from the dendrites, the positive and negative ions are effectively added in summation, by simple virtue of being mixed together in the solution inside the cell's body.

- *Axon* – The axon gets its signal from the summation behavior which occurs inside the soma. The opening to the axon essentially samples the electrical potential of the solution inside the soma. Once the soma reaches a certain potential, the axon will transmit an all-in signal pulse down its length. In this regard, the axon behaves as the ability for us to connect our artificial neuron to other artificial neurons.

Unlike most artificial neurons, however, biological neurons fire in discrete pulses. Each time the electrical potential inside the soma reaches a certain threshold, a pulse is transmitted down the axon. This pulsing can be translated into continuous values. The rate (activations per second, etc.) at which an axon fires converts directly into the rate at which neighboring cells get signal ions introduced into them. The faster a biological neuron fires, the faster nearby neurons accumulate electrical potential (or lose electrical potential, depending on the "weighting" of the dendrite that connects to the neuron that fired). It is this conversion that allows computer scientists and mathematicians to simulate biological neural networks using artificial neurons which can output distinct values (often from –1 to 1).

History

The first artificial neuron was the Threshold Logic Unit (TLU), or Linear Threshold Unit, first proposed by Warren McCulloch and Walter Pitts in 1943. The model was specifically targeted as a computational model of the "nerve net" in the brain. As a transfer function, it employed a threshold, equivalent to using the Heaviside step function. Initially, only a simple model was considered, with binary inputs and outputs, some restrictions on the possible weights, and a more flexible threshold value. Since the beginning it was already noticed that any boolean function could be implemented by networks of such devices, what is easily seen from the fact that one can implement the AND and OR functions, and use them in the disjunctive or the conjunctive normal form. Researchers also soon realized that cyclic networks, with feedbacks through neurons, could define dynamical systems with memory, but most of the research concentrated (and still does) on strictly feed-forward networks because of the smaller difficulty they present.

One important and pioneering artificial neural network that used the linear threshold function was the perceptron, developed by Frank Rosenblatt. This model already considered more flexible weight values in the neurons, and was used in machines with adaptive capabilities. The representation of the threshold values as a bias term was introduced by Bernard Widrow in 1960.

In the late 1980s, when research on neural networks regained strength, neurons with more continuous shapes started to be considered. The possibility of differentiating the activation function allows the direct use of the gradient descent and other optimization algorithms for the adjustment of the weights. Neural networks also started to be used as a general function approximation model. The best known training algorithm called backpropagation has been rediscovered several times but its first development goes back to the work of Paul Werbos.

Types of Transfer Functions

The transfer function of a neuron is chosen to have a number of properties which either enhance or simplify the network containing the neuron. Crucially, for instance, any multilayer perceptron using a *linear* transfer function has an equivalent single-layer network; a non-linear function is therefore necessary to gain the advantages of a multi-layer network.

Below, u refers in all cases to the weighted sum of all the inputs to the neuron, i.e. for n inputs,

$$u = \sum_{i=1}^{n} w_i x_i$$

where w is a vector of *synaptic weights* and **x** is a vector of inputs.

Step Function

The output y of this transfer function is binary, depending on whether the input meets a specified threshold, θ. The "signal" is sent, i.e. the output is set to one, if the activation meets the threshold.

$$y = \begin{cases} 1 & \text{if } u \geq \theta \\ 0 & \text{if } u < \theta \end{cases}$$

This function is used in perceptrons and often shows up in many other models. It performs a division of the space of inputs by a hyperplane. It is specially useful in the last layer of a network intended to perform binary classification of the inputs. It can be approximated from other sigmoidal functions by assigning large values to the weights.

Linear Combination

In this case, the output unit is simply the weighted sum of its inputs plus a *bias* term. A number of such linear neurons perform a linear transformation of the input vector. This is usually more useful in the first layers of a network. A number of analysis tools exist based on linear models, such as harmonic analysis, and they can all be used in neural networks with this linear neuron. The bias term allows us to make affine transformations to the data.

Sigmoid

A fairly simple non-linear function, the sigmoid function such as the logistic function also has an easily calculated derivative, which can be important when calculating the weight updates in the network. It thus makes the network more easily manipulable mathematically, and was attractive to early computer scientists who needed to minimize the computational load of their simulations.

It was previously commonly seen in multilayer perceptrons. However, recent work has shown sigmoid neurons to be less effective than rectified linear neurons. The reason is that the gradients computed by the backpropagation algorithm tend to diminish towards zero as activations propagate through layers of sigmoidal neurons, making it difficult to optimize neural networks using multiple layers of sigmoidal neurons.

Pseudocode Algorithm

The following is a simple pseudocode implementation of a single TLU which takes boolean inputs (true or false), and returns a single boolean output when activated. An object-oriented model is used. No method of training is defined, since several exist. If a purely functional model were used, the class TLU below would be replaced with a function TLU with input parameters threshold, weights, and inputs that returned a boolean value.

```
class TLU defined as:

 data member threshold : number

 data member weights : list of numbers of size X

 function member fire( inputs : list of booleans of size X ) : boolean defined as:

  variable T : number

  T ← 0

  for each i in 1 to X :

   if inputs(i) is true :

    T ← T + weights(i)

   end if

  end for each

  if T > threshold :

   return true

  else:

   return false

  end if

 end function

end class
```

Limitations

Simple artificial neurons, such as the McCulloch–Pitts model, are sometimes described as "caricature models", since they are intended to reflect one or more neurophysiological observations, but without regard to realism.

Comparison with Biological Neuron Coding

Research has shown that unary coding is used in the neural circuits responsible for birdsong production. The use of unary in biological networks is presumably due to the inherent simplicity of the coding. Another contributing factor could be that unary coding provides a certain degree of error correction.

Hodgkin-Huxley Model

The Hodgkin-Huxley model explains how the dynamics of ion channels (Na+, K+ etc) contribute to the generation of an Action Potential in a neuron.

An Action Potential is a sharp voltage spike elicited by stimulating a neuron with a current that exceeds a certain threshold value. The current amplitude is increased gradually, at a threshold amplitude, the voltage response does not increase proportionally. It shows a sharp, disproportionate increase. Once the membrane voltage reaches a threshold value, it increase further rapidly to maximum value and drops again rapidly to a value that is less than resting value, before returning to the baseline value after a delay.

To describe the processes that lead to the generation of an AP from the introduction on Nernst Potential, we present a simple ion channel model which expresses how the channel conductance contributes to the membrane potential, and conversely, in case of voltage-sensitive channels, how the membrane potential controls channel conductance. Finally we place the above components in a full circuit model of neural membrane - the Hodgkin-Huxley model.

Now let us calculate the typical values of Nernst potentials of Na+ and K+ for a neuron.

Nernst Potential

Sodium Nernst Potential

Under resting conditions sodium concentration outside the neuron $\left([Na+]_o\right)$ equals 440 mM, while inside $\left(\left([Na+]_i\right)\right)$ it is 60 mM. From eqn. we calculate Na+ Nernst potential $\left(E_{Na}\right)$ to be about 50 mV.

Potassium Nernst potential:

Similarly under resting conditions, $\left[K+\right]_o$ equals 20 mM, while [K+]i is 400 mM. Therefore, E_K is about -77 mV.

The Nernst potentials, like the membrane potential, are always measured inside, with the extracellular space as the reference. Also note that Na+ Nernst potential is positive inside, and K+ Nernst potential is negative inside. In addition to Nernst potential, an ion channel also has a conductance, which is higher when it is in OPEN state than when it is closed. Channel conductance is usually expressed not in 'per channel' terms, but the total conductance of a whole patch of the membrane containing that channel, expressed in 'Siemens/area'. Thus, again under resting conditions, Na+ conductance is about 120 mS/cm2 and K+ conductance is about 36mS/cm2.

Modeling the Neural Membrane

Electrical response of a neuron depends on the ion channels present and the membrane itself. Once we know the Nernst potential associated with a channel and the channel conductance we are in a position to build a basic model of an ion channel. The model is meant to capture the voltage-current (V-I) characteristics of the ion channel. Since a battery (Nernst potential) and a conductance are associated with the channel, we can represent the channel in of the following two ways: the battery in series (or parallel) with the conductance. Let us determine which of the two are correct. When the conductance is 0, as when the channel is closed, current through the channel is 0, irrespective of the value of the Nernst potential. This rule is satisfied only when the battery and conductance are in series and not in parallel. Therefore, as a first cut we represent an ion channel as a series of a battery and a conductance.

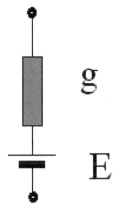

A basic model of an ion channel

Since there are a variety of ion channels with distinct values of E and g, we have a separate branch for each of them. All these branches must be connected in parallel since all the channels stagger across the membrane, and share the same membrane voltage. In addition to the ion channels, the membrane itself is another electrical component that controls the dynamics of the membrane potential. The neural membrane is a lipid bilayer with insulating properties. Due to its bilayer structure, the membrane is modeled as a parallel plate capacitor. Thus the various ion channels and the membrane together may be depicted as an electrical equivalent circuit as follows:

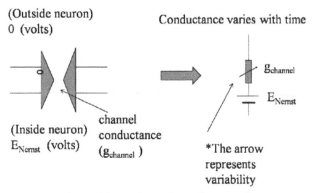

An ion channel has voltage dependant conductance

Now if all the circuit components (capacitance, conductances, batteries) are time-invariant, then all the branches corresponding to ion channels can be combined into a single equivalent branch consisting of a single conductance and a battery. This can be done by invoking a well-known result from electrical engineering known as Thevenin's theorem. With such simplification a model of the membrane looks as shown in figure.

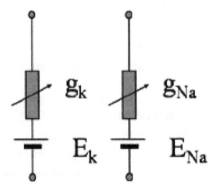

$$E_L = 10.6 \text{ mV}$$
$$g_L = 0.3 \text{mS/cm}^2$$

Resultant branch equivalent for time invariant branches, corresponding to ion channels

This is a simple, linear RC circuit and is not likely to exhibit the interesting voltage dynamics underlying AP generation, which is basically a nonlinear behavior. The root cause of AP behavior is presence of voltage-dependent ion channels, which may be regarded as nonlinear conductances since their conductance depends on membrane voltage. Particularly voltage- dependent Na^+ and K^+ channels play a crucial role in AP generation. These are shown in Figure.

Circuit equivalents for sodium and potassium channels

We now take up the question of modeling a general voltage-sensitive channel first, followed by specific models for voltage-sensitive Na^+ and K^+ channels.

A General Model of a Voltage-sensitive Channel

Mathematical treatment of voltage dependent gating of channels has two parts. First, we describe the dynamics of switching between open/close states. This description is kept general, without reference to a specific gating mechanism. Next, we describe voltage-gating, or, the manner in which switching dynamics is influenced by membrane voltage.

Channel Switching

When we set out to describe switching between open and closed states of channel there is an implicit assumption that the channel has only two states. This assumption is not true. Complex channels do have a large number of intermediate states that are not strictly 'open' or 'closed.' Channel switching in those cases involves switching among all those states. But for the moment we consider only simple channels with only two states – open and closed.

Channel switching can described as a unimolecular chemical reaction where a molecule – the channel protein – switches between two states in figure.

$$C_c \;\underset{k^-}{\overset{k^+}{\rightleftharpoons}}\; C_o$$

Channel Switching

where C_c and C_o denote the channel in open and closed states, and k^+ and k^- are the forward and reverse rate coefficients. If x is the fraction of the channels in open state, and (1-x) is the fraction of channels in closed state, dynamics of state transition may be described as a first order chemical reaction as follows:

$$\frac{dx}{dt} = k^- x - k^+ (1-x)$$

The above equation can also be written as,

$$\tau \frac{dx}{dt} = -x + x_\infty$$

where,

$$x_\infty = \frac{k^+}{k^+ + k^-}$$

$$\tau_\infty = \frac{1}{k^+ + k^-}$$

Note that the above simple description is applicable for a statistical ensemble of channels. Since a cell membrane typically has a few thousand ion channels the above description is justified. Switching behavior in single channels, which can be measured using techniques like patch- clamping, is far more complex. Since our objective is to study membrane voltage changes it is sufficient to treat channels as an ensemble.

Complete solution of eqn. requires knowledge of K^+ and K^-. In voltage- sensitive channels these quantities are functions of membrane voltage and that is the mechanism by which membrane voltage controls channel gating.

Since ion channels are proteins which contain charged amino acid side chains, membrane potential can influence the rate of open/close transitions. Using Arrhenius expressions, the rate constants can be expressed in terms of the membrane potential as:

$$k^+ = k_0^+ \exp(-\alpha V) \qquad and \qquad k^- = k_0^- \exp(-\beta V)$$

where k_0^+ and k_0^- are independent of membrane voltage.

Substituting the above formulae for k_0^+ and k_0^- in eqn. above, we have

$$x_\infty = \frac{1}{1 + \left(k_0^- / k_0^+\right)\exp\left((\alpha - \beta)V\right)}$$

$$\tau = \frac{1}{k_0^+ \exp(-\alpha V)} \frac{1}{1 + \left(k_0^- / k_0^+\right)\exp\left((\alpha - \beta)V\right)}$$

Now let us define,

$$S_0 = \frac{1}{(\beta - \alpha)} \qquad and \qquad V_0 = \frac{\ln\left(k_0^- / k_0^+\right)}{(\beta - \alpha)}$$

Substituting S_0 and V_0 in eqns. (3.3.1.5, 3.3.1.6) we obtain,

$$x_\infty = \frac{1}{1 + \exp\left(-(V - V_0)/S_0\right)}$$

$$\tau = \frac{\exp(\alpha V)}{k_0^+}\left(\frac{1}{1 + \exp\left(-(V - V_0)/S_0\right)}\right)$$

Using hyperbolic functions, the last two expressions can be rewritten as,

$$x_\infty = 0.5\left(1 + \tanh\left((V - V_0)/(2S_0)\right)\right)$$

$$\tau = \frac{\exp\left(V(\alpha + \beta)/2\right)}{2\sqrt{k_0^+ k_0^-}\left(-(V - V_0)/S_0\right)}$$

Eqn. tells us how many channels are open once the entire population of channels comes to equilibrium at a given steady state membrane voltage. Figure depicts the dependence of open probability (x) on membrane voltage for various values of V_0 and S_0. If S_0 is positive, channels open with increasing membrane voltages. Such gates are known as activation gates. When S_0 is negative, gates close with increasing membrane voltages. Such gates are known as inactivation gates. V_0 determines the voltage at which the transition from 'mostly open' to 'mostly closed' takes place.

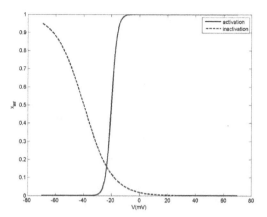

The effect of membrane voltage (V) on x_∞

The solid line corresponds to an activation gate ($S_0 = 2$) and the dashed line corresponds to an in-activation gate ($S_0 = -10$). Note the smaller the magnitude of S_0, the steeper the curve. V_0 for the activation and inactivation gates are -20 mV and -40 mV respectively.

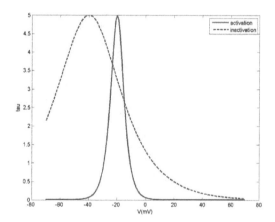

Effect of membrane voltage on the time constant of relaxation (t).

For the two curves shown in figure, it is assumed that $\alpha+\beta = 0$, and

$$\phi = \frac{1}{2\sqrt{k_0^+ k_0^-}}, where\ 2\sqrt{k_0^+ k_0^-} = 0.2\text{ms}^{-1}$$

In figure, for the solid line, $S_0 = 2$; $V_0 = -20$, whereas for the dotted line, $S_0 = 10$; $V_0 = -40$. Note that the sign of S_0 does not affect t since it is an even function of S_0. V_0 denotes the voltage at which t is maximum. The magnitude of S_0 determines the sharpness of the peak.

Channel Gating

In the above account of channel switching we have given the impression that there is a single "bottle-neck" in the pore which closes the channel. However, such a description is not completely accurate. There can be several local "bottle-necks," simply referred to as gates, which can control channel closure.

To describe channel switching then we must be able to express the kinetics of all the gates in the channel. The question now is to describe the dynamics of single gates – the gate kinetics – and express the switching of the whole channel in terms of the component gates.

Our work is made easy by the fact that gate kinetics is also treated just as we have treated channel switching in eqns. If we consider only channels with single gates, equations for gate kinetics would looks identical to eqns. with the only difference that 'x' now represents the fraction of open gates, which is also interpreted as probability of the gate being in open state. The same quantity is also called the gating variable. Since we are considering at the moment channels with only a single gate, fraction of open channels is the same as fraction of open gates.

Channels with multiple gates:

If a channel has K gates, with open probabilities of the gates denoted, by x_1, x_2, x_K, then the open probability, denoted by x, of the entire channel is given as:

$x = x_1 * x_2 * ... x_K$ since the channel is open only when all the gates are open.

Modeling a Voltage-dependent Na⁺ Channel

The voltage-dependent Na⁺ channel in the Hodgkin-Huxley model is thought to have 4 gates – three of them being activation gates, and the last one being an inactivation gate. The three activation gates are thought to be identical, denoted by a common gating variable, m. The

inactivation gate is denoted by the gating variable h. Thus the open probability of the entire gate is m³ h. If the conductance of a population of Na⁺ channels in which all Na⁺ channels are fully open is g_{Na}^{max} then the conductance, g_{Na} of the population in general conditions (some Na⁺ channels are closed) is,

$$g_{Na} = g_{Na}^{max} m^3 h$$

The gate kinetics of m variables may be described as,

$$\frac{dm}{dt} = \alpha_m (V_m)(1-m) - \beta_m (V_m) m$$

Alternatively, the above equation may be written in the form in terms of the time constant and steady state value of the gating variable m. But the form of eqn. above is more commonly used in literature. Similarly, the gate kinetics of h variable may be written as,

$$\frac{dh}{dt} = \alpha_h (V_m)(1-h) - \beta_h (V_m) h$$

Modeling a Voltage-dependent K⁺ channel

The voltage-dependent K⁺ channel used in the HH model is thought to have 4 identical activation gates, denoted by the gating variable n. Thus the open probability of the entire gate is n^4. If the conductance of a population of K⁺ channels in which all K⁺ channels are fully open is g_K^{max} then the conductance, g_K, of the population is,

$$g_K = g_{K^{max}} n^4$$

Dynamics of the gating variable, n, is expressed as,

$$\frac{dn}{dt} = \alpha_n(V_m)(1-n) - \beta_n(V_m)n$$

The alpha and beta functions $(\alpha_m, \beta_m \; \alpha_n, \beta_n \; \alpha_h, \beta_h)$ are estimated from voltage clamp experiments.

The Hodgkin-Huxley Model

With this background, we are ready to introduce the Hodgkin-Huxley model equations. To this end, we redraw the circuit of fig. with a slight modification. In the circuit of figure, we have combined all the ion channels using the Thevenin's theorem. However, such compression is possible only when the all the components (conductances and batteries) are constant. But since conductances of voltage-sensitive channels vary through time, such compression is invalid. Thus we have to maintain the distinctness of voltage-sensitive Na⁺ and K⁺ channels. All the remaining channels, which are voltage-independent, can still be compressed to a single branch, consisting of a conductance and battery. This branch is thought to represent a notional ion channel that is equivalent to the sum total of all the voltage-independent ion channels in the membrane. This ion channel is called a 'leakage channel' since it is constantly open, allowing 'leakage' of current from the neuron. We thus have four branches in the circuit: the capacitor, the voltage-sensitive Na⁺ channel, the voltage-sensitive Na⁺ channel and the leakage channel. External current, I_{ext}, applied to the neuron can be split into four components:

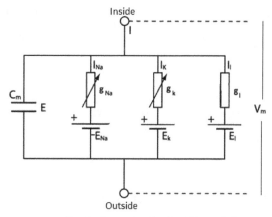

Equivalent circuit of a HH model

$$I_{ext} = I_C + I_{Na} + I_K + I_l$$

I_C current through the capacitance

I_{Na} - current through the Na⁺ channel

I_K – current through the K⁺ channel

I_l – current through the leakage conductance

The above current equation may be expanded as,

$$C\frac{dV_m}{dt}+g_{Na}\left(V_m-E_{Na}\right)+g_K\left(V_m-E_K\right)+g_l\left(V_m-E_l\right)=I_{ext}$$

or

$$C\frac{dV_m}{dt}=-g_{Na}^{max}m^3h\left(V_m-E_{Na}\right)-g_K^{max}n^4\left(V_m-E_K\right)-g_l\left(V_m-E_l\right)+I_{ext}$$

The above equation that describes membrane voltage dynamics must be supplemented by the following equations to complete the definition of the Hodgkin-Huxley model.

$$\frac{dm}{dt}=\alpha_m\left(V_m\right)\left(1-m\right)-\beta_m\left(V_m\right)m$$

$$\frac{dh}{dt}=\alpha_h\left(V_m\right)\left(1-h\right)-\beta_h\left(V_m\right)h$$

$$\frac{dn}{dt}=\alpha_n\left(V_m\right)\left(1-n\right)-\beta_n\left(V_m\right)h$$

$$g_{Na}=g_{Na^{max}}m^3h$$

$$g_K=g_K^{max}n^4$$

$$\alpha_n=\frac{0.01\left(v_m+50\right)}{\left\{1-\exp\left(-\frac{\left[v_m+50\right]}{10}\right)\right\}},\ \beta_n=0.125\exp\left(-\frac{\left[v_m+60\right]}{80}\right)$$

$$\alpha_m=\frac{0.1\left(v_m+35.0\right)}{\left\{1-\exp\left(-\frac{\left[v_m+35\right]}{10}\right)\right\}},\ \beta_m=4\exp\left(-0.0556\left[v_m+60\right]\right)$$

$$\alpha_m=0.07\exp\left(-0.05\left[v_m+60\right]\right),\ \beta_h=\frac{1}{\left(1+\exp\left\{-0.1\left[v_m+30\right]\right\}\right)}$$

Dependencies among the variables involved in the HH model are depicted in figure.

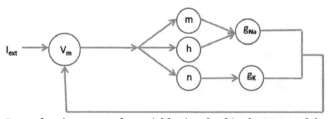

Dependencies among the variables involved in the HH model

The Voltage, Conductances, gating variables vs. time for different I values showing various dynamics have been simulated below. Figure shows the complete frequency dynamics of the HH model.

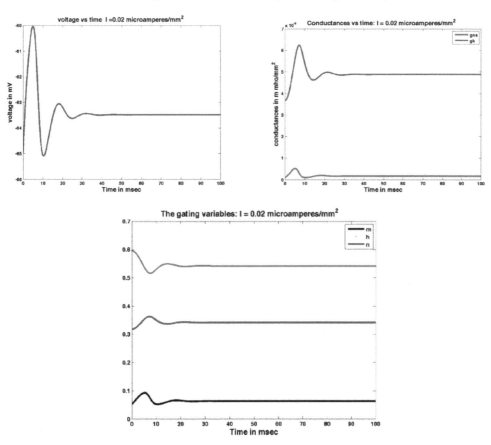

Voltage vs. time; Conductances vs. time; gating variables vs. time for I = 0.02μA/mm²

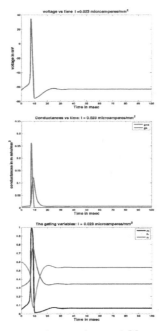

Voltage vs. time; Conductances vs. time;gating variables vs. time for I = 0.023μA/mm²

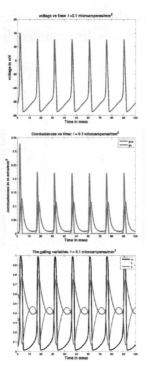

Voltage vs. time; Conductances vs. time; gating variables vs. time for I = 0.1μA/mm²

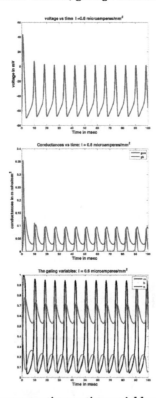

Voltage vs. time; Conductances vs. time;gating variables vs. time for I = 0.6μA/mm²

The HH model Action potential dynamics see the following fixed points. Before I1, no AP's are seen. Between I1 and I2, finite number of Action potentials are seen, and between I2 and I3, Limit cycle behavior is noticed. After I3, no Action potentials are seen.

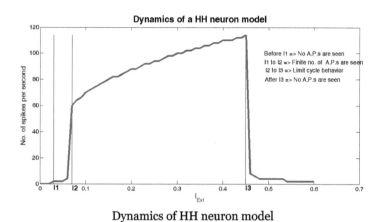

Dynamics of HH neuron model

Code

%THIS PROGRAM DEMONSTRATES HODGKIN HUXLEY MODEL IN CURRENT CLAMP EXPERIMENTS AND SHOWS ACTION POTENTIAL PROPAGATION

%Time is in msecs, voltage in mvs, conductances in m mho/mm^2, capacitance in microF/mm^2

% threshold value of current is 0.0223

k=1;

istep=0.01;

forImpCur=0:istep:0.6

%TimeTot=input('enter the time for which stimulus is applied in milliseconds');

gkmax=.36;

vk=-77;

gnamax=1.20;

vna=50; gl=0.003;

vl=-54.387;

cm=.01;

dt=0.01;

niter=50000;

t=(1:niter)*dt;

iapp=ImpCur*ones(1,niter);

%for i=1:100

%   iapp(1,i)=ImpCur;

```
%end;
v=-64.9964;
 m=0.0530;
 h=0.5960;
n=0.3177;
gnahist=zeros(1,niter);
gkhist=zeros(1,niter);
vhist=zeros(1,niter);
mhist=zeros(1,niter);
hhist=zeros(1,niter);
nhist=zeros(1,niter);
foriter=1:niter
gna=gnamax*m^3*h;
gk=gkmax*n^4;
 gtot=gna+gk+gl;
vinf = ((gna*vna+gk*vk+gl*vl)+ iapp(iter))/gtot;
tauv = cm/gtot;
v=vinf+(v-vinf)*exp(-dt/tauv);
alpham = 0.1*(v+40)/(1-exp(-(v+40)/10));
betam = 4*exp(-0.0556*(v+65));
alphan = 0.01*(v+55)/(1-exp(-(v+55)/10));
betan = 0.125*exp(-(v+65)/80);
alphah = 0.07*exp(-0.05*(v+65));
betah = 1/(1+exp(-0.1*(v+35)));
taum = 1/(alpham+betam);
tauh = 1/(alphah+betah);
taun = 1/(alphan+betan);
 minf = alpham*taum;
```

```
hinf = alphah*tauh;

ninf = alphan*taun;

m=minf+(m-minf)*exp(-dt/taum);

h=hinf+(h-hinf)*exp(-dt/tauh);

n=ninf+(n-ninf)*exp(-dt/taun);

vhist(iter)=v;

mhist(iter)=m;

 hhist(iter)=h;

nhist(iter)=n;

gnahist(iter) = gna;

gkhist(iter) = gk;

 end

j=1;

realpeaks=zeros;

[peaks, locs]=findpeaks(vhist);

for temp=1:length(peaks)

if peaks(temp) >=10 % minimum value at which a waveform is considered AP. realpeaks(j)=peaks(-temp);

j=j+1;

end;

end;

ifrealpeaks ~= 0 no_of_peaks(k)=length(realpeaks);

else

no_of_peaks(k)=0;

 end;

k=k+1 end;

figure(1)

%subplot(2,1,1)
```

```
plot(t,vhist)

title('voltage vs time')

figure(2)

%subplot(2,1,2)

plot(t,mhist,'y-', t,hhist,'g.',t,nhist,'b-')

 legend('m','h','n')

figure(3)

gna=gnamax*(mhist.^3).*hhist;

gk=gkmax*nhist.^4;

clf plot(t,gna,'r');

holdon

plot(t,gk,'b');

legend('gna','gk')

holdoff

figure(4);

X=0:istep:0.6;

plot(X,no_of_peaks*1000/(niter/100));

 xlabel('I_{Ext}');

ylabel('No. of spikes per second')

holdon;

for l=2:length(no_of_peaks) %to define I1, I2, I3.

 ifno_of_peaks(l)>0 &&no_of_peaks(l-1)==0

I1=(l-1)*istep

end;

ifno_of_peaks(l)>no_of_peaks(l-1)+4

I2=(l-1)*istep

end;

ifno_of_peaks(l)<no_of_peaks(l-1)-2
```

I3=(l-2)*istep

end;

end;

I1=0*no_of_peaks*1000/(niter/100)+I1; plot(I1,no_of_peaks*1000/(niter/100),'r');

 text(I1(1),-3,'I1');

I2=0*no_of_peaks*1000/(niter/100)+I2; plot(I2,no_of_peaks*1000/(niter/100),'g');

 text(I2(1),-3,'I2');

I3=0*no_of_peaks*1000/(niter/100)+I3; plot(I3,no_of_peaks*1000/(niter/100),'y');

text(I3(1),-3,'I3');

text(0.5,100,'Before I1 => No A.P.s are seen');

text(0.5,95,'I1 to I2 => Finite no. of   A.P.s are seen');

text(0.5,90,'I2 to I3 => Infinite no.of A.P.s are seen');

text(0.5,85,'After I3 => No A.P.s are seen');

FitzHugh–Nagumo Model

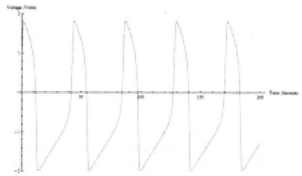

Graph of v with parameters I=0.5, a=0.7, b=0.8, and τ=12.5

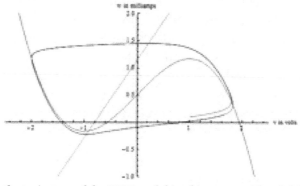

The blue line is the trajectory of the FHN model in phase space. The pink line is the cubic nullcline and the yellow line is the linear nullcline.

The FitzHugh–Nagumo model (FHN), named after Richard FitzHugh (1922 – 2007) who suggested the system in 1961 and J. Nagumo *et al.* who created the equivalent circuit the following year, describes a prototype of an excitable system (e.g., a neuron).

The FHN Model is an example of a relaxation oscillator because, if the external stimulus I_{ext} exceeds a certain threshold value, the system will exhibit a characteristic excursion in phase space, before the variables v and w relax back to their rest values.

This behaviour is typical for spike generations (a short, nonlinear elevation of membrane voltage v, diminished over time by a slower, linear recovery variable w) in a neuron after stimulation by an external input current.

The equations for this dynamical system read

$$\dot{v} = v - \frac{v^3}{3} - w + I_{ext}$$

$$\tau \dot{w} = v + a - bw.$$

The dynamics of this system can be nicely described by zapping between the left and right branch of the cubic nullcline.

The FitzHugh–Nagumo model is a simplified version of the Hodgkin–Huxley model which models in a detailed manner activation and deactivation dynamics of a spiking neuron. In the original papers of FitzHugh, this model was called Bonhoeffer–van der Pol oscillator (named after Karl Friedrich Bonhoeffer and Balthasar van der Pol) because it contains the van der Pol oscillator as a special case for $a = b = 0$. The equivalent circuit was suggested by Jin-ichi Nagumo, Suguru Arimoto, and Shuji Yoshizawa.

Simplified Neuron Models

We have introduced the HH model which is the earliest model of action potential (AP) generation in an axon. It shows how voltage-sensitive dynamics of sodium and potassium channels results in generation of APs. But real neurons have a much large variety of ion channels. There are dozens of voltage- and Ca2+-gated channels known today. Combinations of these channels can give rise to an astronomically large number of neuron models. Even the HH model, the simplest model of AP generation that we encountered so far, has 4 differential equations, three of them being nonlinear. More realistic neuron models with larger number of ion channels can easily become mathematically untractable. It would be desirable to construct simplified models, with fewer variables, and milder nonlinearities, in such a way that the reduced model preserves the essential dynamics of their more complex versions. One of the first reduced model of that kind is the Fitzhugh-Nagumo neuron model.

FitzHugh-Nagumo model is a two-variable neuron model, constructed by reducing the 4-variable HH model, by applying suitable assumptions.

Hodgkin- Huxley model:

$$C\frac{dv}{dt}+\bar{g}_{Na}m^3h\left(v-E_{Na}\right)+\bar{g}_k n^4\left(v-E_k\right)+g_L\left(v-E_L\right)=I_{at}$$

$$\frac{dm}{dt}=\alpha_m\left(V_m\right)\left(1-m\right)-\beta_m\left(V_m\right)m$$

$$\frac{dh}{dt}=\alpha_h\left(V_m\right)\left(1-h\right)-\beta_h\left(V_m\right)h$$

$$\frac{dn}{dt}=\alpha_n\left(V_m\right)\left(1-n\right)-\beta_n\left(V_m\right)n$$

Assumptions:-

The time scales for m, h and n variables are not all of the same order. These disparities provide a basis for eliminating some of the gating variables.

1) Since the time scale for m is much smaller than that of the other two, we assume that m relaxes faster than the other two gating variables. Therefore, we let,

$$\frac{dm}{dt}=0 \text{ i.e.,}$$

$$\frac{dm}{dt}=\alpha_m\left(v\right)\left(1-m\right)-\beta_m\left(v\right)m$$

$$0=\alpha_m\left(v\right)-\left(\alpha_m\left(v\right)+\beta_m\left(v\right)\right)\left(m\right)$$

$$m=\frac{\alpha_m\left(v\right)}{\alpha_m\left(v\right)+\beta_m\left(v\right)}$$

2) h varies too slowly. Therefore, we let h to be a constant, $h=h_0$

The resulting system has only two variables (v, n). After transformation to dimensionless variables, and some approximations, the resulting FN model may be defined as,

$$\frac{dv}{dt}=f\left(v\right)-w+I_m$$

where $f\left(v\right)=v\left(a-v\right)\left(v-1\right)$

$$\frac{dw}{dt}=bv-rw$$

In the above system, v is analogous to the membrane voltage, and w represents all the three gating variables.

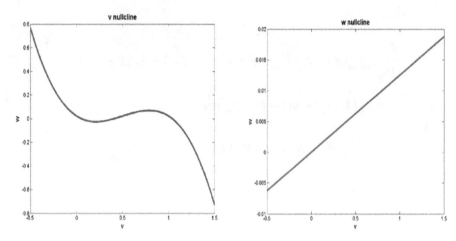

The nullclines V and w

The two nullclines of the above system are,

$$F(v,w) \equiv f(v) - w + I_a = 0 \quad \text{(F-nullcline)}$$
$$g(v,w) \equiv bv - rw = 0 \quad \text{(g-nullcline)}$$

To examine the stability of a stationary point, we calculate the Jacobian, A, of the system at that point.

$$A = \begin{bmatrix} \dfrac{\partial F}{\partial v} & \dfrac{\partial F}{\partial \omega} \\ \dfrac{\partial g}{\partial v} & \dfrac{\partial g}{\partial \omega} \end{bmatrix} = \begin{bmatrix} f'(v) & -1 \\ b & -r \end{bmatrix}$$

$$\tau = f'(v) - r$$

$$\Delta = f'(v)(-r)$$

The type of the stationary point can be expressed in terms of determinant, Δ, and trace, τ, of the Jacobian, using the following rules:

-if $\Delta < 0$, the stationary point is a saddle irrespective of the value of τ .

-if $\Delta > 0$, $\tau < 0$, stable point

-if $\Delta > 0$, $\tau > 0$, unstable point.

$$\Delta >$$
$$f(v)(-r) > -b$$
$$f(v)r \quad b$$
$$f(v) \quad -$$

That is, $\Delta > 0$, when the slope of the F-nullcline is lesser than slope of w-nullcline.

$$\tau > 0, \Rightarrow f'(v) - r > 0$$
$$\Rightarrow f'(v) > 0 \quad (approx)$$

Now let us consider the behavior of FN model as external current I_a is gradually increased.

$I_a = 0$ Excitability

The phase-plane shown below depicts the situation when $I_a = 0$. There is only one stationary point at the origin.

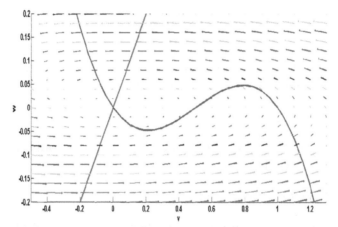

Phase plane analysis: Excitability at a=0.5; b=0.1; r=0.1; $I_a = 0$

Stability of origin:

a) Slope of F-nullcline> slope of w-nullcline $\Delta > 0$

b) $f'(v) < 0, \Rightarrow \tau < 0$ ∴ Origin is stable.

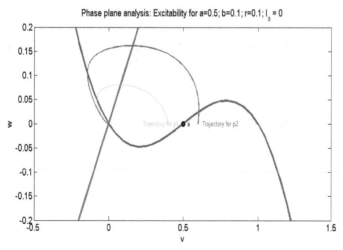

The points a,p1,p2 and their trajectories

Consider the evolution of the variable v (membrane voltage) when the initial condition is at points p1 or p2.

This behavior will first be anticipated using loose arguments, and then confirmed using simulations.

The F- and w-nullclines in fig. above intersect only at one point (the origin) and therefore divide the plane into four regions, numbered from 1 to 4. The flow patterns in the four regions can be seen to be as follows:

Region 1: $\dot{v} < 0, \dot{w} > 0$

Region 2: $\dot{v} < 0, \dot{w} < 0$

Region 3: $\dot{v} > 0, \dot{w} < 0$

Region 4: $\dot{v} > 0, \dot{w} < 0$

We have just talked about the signs of $\dot{v}, \dot{w}$, but it must be noted that, far from the null- clines, the magnitude of $\dot{w}$ is much smaller than that of $\dot{v}$, since b,r<<1.

We divide the F-null-cline into three segments: Segment 1 (to the left of point M),

Segment 2 (between points M and N) and Segment 3 (to the right of point N). We will refer to these segments in the following discussion.

Let us now consider the two initial conditions:

Initial condition at p1: This point is inside region 1. Therefore the flow is leftwards, with a small upward component. The system state approaches the origin and settles there, confirming our earlier result that the origin is the only stable point.

Initial condition at p2: This point is inside region 4, where the flow is rightwards with a small upward component. Therefore the system state moves rightwards until it hits the F- nullcline inside Segment 3. Since the flow has no horizontal component on the F- nullcline, the small upward component pushes the state upwards. In Segment 3 of F- nullcine there is a tendency for the state stay on the F-nullcline, since the flow is leftwards on its right, and rightwards on its left. Therefore, the state creeps along the F- nullcline in the upward direction until it reaches the topmost point, N, on the F-nullcline. Beyond this point the flow is still upwards and leftwards while the F-nullcline bends downwards. Therefore, the state leaves the F-nullcline and drifts leftwards until it reaches Segment 1. The situation now similar to what we encountered on Segment 3, but with a downward flow component. Therefore the state creeps downward along Segment 3 until reaches the origin where it finally settles down.

Therefore, when p2 is the initial condition, the system exhibits this large excursion by which the membrane voltage reaches a maximum before it returns to the origin. Such an excursion of membrane voltage resembles an action potentials.

Therefore the FitzHugh-Nagumo neuron model exhibits excitability. For the initial membrane less than a threshold value (=a), the voltage quickly returns to zero. When the initial voltage exceeds the threshold (=a), the voltage exhibits an action potential.

p1 , p2 $\Rightarrow$ Initial voltages $v(0)$

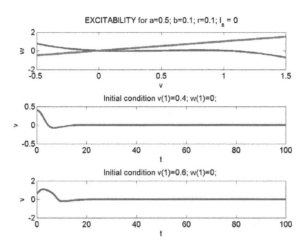

a) The nullclines v and w, and 'v' simulation from b) p1 and c) p2

Limit Cycles ($I_a > 0$):

As I_a increases, for a range of values of I_a, the w-nullcline intersections the F-nullcline in the "middle branch" where the F-nullcline has a positive slope. In this case too there only a single intersection.

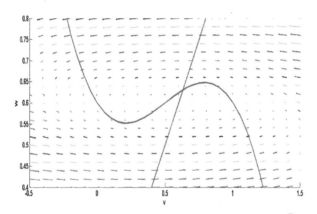

Phase plane analysis: Oscillations at a=0.5; b=0.1; r=0.1; I_a =0.6

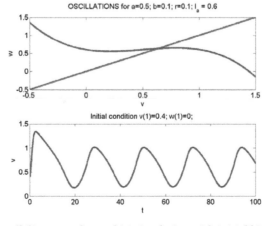

a) The nullclines v and w and 'v' simulation with initial b) v(1)=0.4

$\tau = f'(v) > 0$ Therefore, the stationary point is unstable.

The rough 'arrowplot' in figure above shows that there is a 'circulating field' around the stationary point, which is unstable. Thus it can be expected that there is a limit cycle enclosing the stationary point, which is actually true. Figure shows the oscillations in membrane voltage (v) produced by a MATLAB program.

Depolarization (Higher I_a):

As I_a increases further, the two nullclines intersect in the "right branch" of the F-nullcline where the slope of F-nullcline is negative.

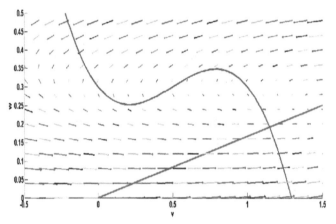

Phase plane analysis: Depolarisation at a=0.5; b=0.1; r=0.6; I_a =0.3

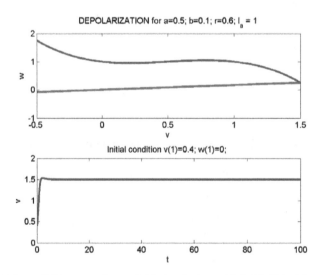

a) The nullclines v and w and 'v' simulation with initial b) v(1)=0.4

Since,

$$f'(v) < \frac{b}{r}, \Delta > 0$$

$$\tau = f'(v) > 0$$

We know that the stationary point is stable. In this case, the membrane voltage remains stable at a high value. This corresponds to regime 4 in the HH model where for a sufficiently high current, the neuron does not fire but remains tonically depolarized.

Bistability

Some real neurons exhibit bistable behavior – their membrane voltage can remain at tonically high ("UP" state) or tonically low ("DOWN" state) values. These UP/DOWN neurons are found in for example in medium spiny neurons of Basal ganglia striatum.

The FN model exhibits bistability for a certain range of model parameters.

Figure below shows a configuration in which the null-clines intersect at three points (p1, p2 and p3). It can easily be shown that p1 and p3 are stable, and p2 is a saddle.

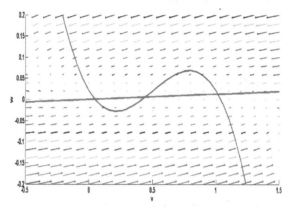

Phase plane analysis: Neuronal on-off bi-stable behavior at a=0.5; b=0.01; r=0.8; I_a =0.02

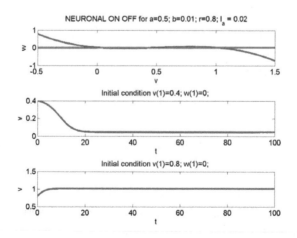

a) The nullclines v and w, and 'v' simulation with initial b) p1: v(1)=0.4 c) p3: v(1) = 0.8

$$@\, p1 : \left(V(1) = 0.4 \right)$$

$$f'(v) < 0 < \frac{b}{r}, \Delta > 0$$

$$\tau = f'(v) < 0, stable$$

$$@\, p2 : \left(V(1) = 0.5 \right)$$

$$f'(v) > \frac{b}{r}, \Delta < 0$$

$$\tau = f'(v) > 0, saddle\, node$$

$$@\, p3 : \left(V(1) = 0.8 \right)$$

$$f'(v) < 0 < \frac{b}{r}, \Delta > 0$$

$$\tau = f'(v) < 0, stable$$

FN model in this case, can remain stable at either p1(low v value, DOWN state) or at p3 (high v value, UP state).

Morris–Lecar Model

The Morris–Lecar model is a biological neuron model developed by Catherine Morris and Harold Lecar to reproduce the variety of oscillatory behavior in relation to Ca^{++} and K^+ conductance in the muscle fiber of the giant barnacle . Morris–Lecar neurons exhibit both class I and class II neuron excitability.

History

Catherine Morris (b. 24 December 1949) is a Canadian biologist. She won a Commonwealth scholarship to study at Cambridge University, where she earned her PhD in 1977. She became a professor at the University of Ottawa in the early 1980s. As of 2015, she is an emeritus professor at the University of Ottawa. Harold Lecar (18 Oct 1935-4 Feb 2014) was an American professor of biophysics and neurobiology at the University of California Berkeley. He graduated with his PhD in physics from Columbia University in 1963.

Experimental Method

The Morris–Lecar experiments relied on the current clamp method established by Keynes *et al.* (1973).

Large specimens of the barnacle *Balanus nubilus* (Pacific Bio-Marine Laboratories Inc., Venice, California) were used. The barnacle was sawed into lateral halves, and the depressor scutorum rostralis muscles were carefully exposed. Individual fibers were dissected, the incision starting from the tendon. The other end of the muscle was cut close to its attachment on the shell and ligatured. Isolated fibers were either used immediately or kept for up to 30 min in standard artificial seawater before use. Experiments were carried out at room temperature of 22 C.

The Principal Assumptions Underlying the Morris–Lecar Model Include

1. Equations apply to a spatially iso-potential patch of membrane. There are two persistent

(non-inactivating) voltage-gated currents with oppositively biased reversal potentials. The depolarizing current is carried by Na+ or Ca2+ ions (or both), depending on the system to be modeled, and the hyperpolarizing current is carried by K+.

2. Activation gates follow changes in membrane potential sufficiently rapidly that the activating conductance can instantaneously relax to its steady-state value at any voltage.

3. The dynamics of the recovery variable can be approximated by a first-order linear differential equation for the probability of channel opening.

Physiological Description

The Morris–Lecar model is a two-dimensional system of nonlinear differential equations. It is considered a simplified model compared to the four-dimensional Hodgkin–Huxley model.

Qualitatively, this system of equations describes the complex relationship between membrane potential and the activation of ion channels within the membrane: the potential depends on the activity of the ion channels, and the activity of the ion channels depends on the voltage. As bifurcation parameters are altered, different classes of neuron behavior are exhibited. τ_N is associated with the relative time scales of the firing dynamics, which varies broadly from cell to cell and exhibits significant temperature dependency.

Quantitatively:

$$C\frac{dV}{dt}=I-g_L(V-V_L)-g_{Ca}M_{ss}(V-V_{Ca})-g_K N(V-V_K)\frac{dN}{dt}=\frac{N_{ss}-N}{\tau_N}$$

$$\frac{dN}{dt}=\frac{N_{ss}-N}{\tau_N}$$

where

$$M_{ss}=\tfrac{1}{2}\cdot(1+\tanh[\tfrac{V-V_1}{V_2}])$$

$$N_{ss}=\tfrac{1}{2}\cdot(1+\tanh[\tfrac{V-V_3}{V_4}])$$

$$\tau_N=1/(\phi\cosh[\tfrac{V-V_3}{2V_4}])$$

Note that the M_{ss} and N_{ss} equations may also be expressed as $M_{ss} = (1 + Exp[-2(V - V_1) / V_2])^{-1}$ and $N_{ss} = (1 + Exp[-2(V - V_3) / V_4])^{-1}$, however most authors prefer the form using the hyperbolic functions.

Variables

- V: membrane potential
- N: recovery variable: the probability that the K+ channel is conducting

Parameters and Constants

- I : applied current
- C : membrane capacitance
- g_L, g_{Ca}, g_K : leak, Ca^{++}, and K$^+$ conductances through membranes channel
- V_L, V_{Ca}, V_K : equilibrium potential of relevant ion channels
- V_1, V_2, V_3, V_4 : tuning parameters for steady state and time constant
- φ : reference frequency

Bifurcations

Bifurcation in the Morris–Lecar model have been analyzed with the applied current I, as the main bifurcation parameter and φ, g_{Ca}, V_3, V_4 as secondary parameters for phase plane analysis.

Possible Bifurcations

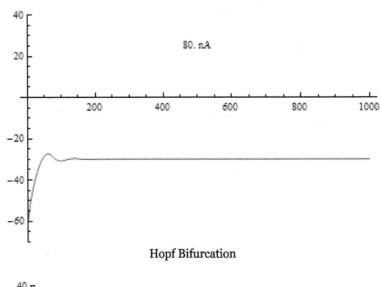

Hopf Bifurcation

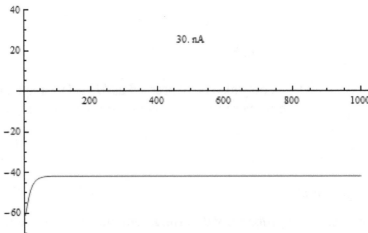

SNIC bifurcation

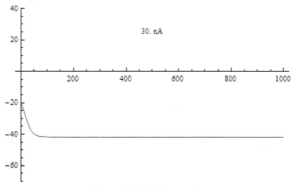

Homoclinic bifurcation

Current clamp simulations of the Morris–Lecar model. The injected current for the SNIC bifurcation and the homoclinic bifurcation is varied between 30 nA and 50 nA, while the current for the Hopf bifurcation is varied between 80nA and 100nA

The Morris-Lecar (ML) model (Morris and Lecar 1981) describes the membrane voltage dynamics of the barnacle muscle fiber. It consists of three channel currents:

    a) A fast activating Ca2$^+$ current (activating variable – m)

    b) A delayed rectifying K$^+$ current (activating variable – w)

    c) A leakage current

Simplifying Assumption:

As in the case of FN model, we assume that the dynamics of m-variable is fast. Therefore, m may be substituted by m_∞

Equations of the ML model are given as,

$$C\frac{dv}{dt} + \bar{g}_{Ca}m_\infty\left(v - E_{Ca}\right) + \bar{g}_k w\left(v - E_k\right) + g_L\left(v - E_L\right) = I_a$$

$$\tau\frac{dw}{dt} = \phi\left(-w + w_\infty\right)$$

$$m_\infty = \frac{1}{2}\left[1 + \tanh\left(\left(v - v_1\right)/v_2\right)\right]$$

$$w_\infty = \frac{1}{2}\left[1 + \tanh\left(\left(v - v_3\right)/v_4\right)\right]$$

$$\tau = 1/\cosh\left(\left(v - v_3\right)/\left(2v_4\right)\right)$$

v-nullcline:

$$w = \frac{I_a - \bar{g}_{Ca}m_\infty\left(v - E_{Ca}\right) - g_L\left(v - E_L\right)}{\bar{g}_k w\left(v - E_k\right)}$$

w-nullcine:

$$w = w_{\infty=} \frac{1}{2}\left[1 + \tanh\left((v - v_3)/v_4\right)\right]$$

Note that the v-nullcline is 'inverted N'-shaped, similar to the F-nullcline of FN model. The w-null-cline has a sigmoidal shape. The v-nullcline can be divided into 'left', 'middle' and 'right' branches. Depending on the branch in which the intersection of V- and w- nullclines, we have different dynamics. The v-nullcine rises with increasing I_a .

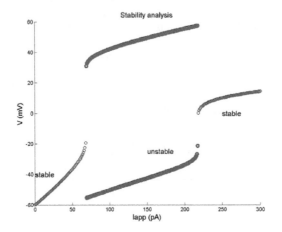

Bifurication plot for the ML model

For I_a in the range (0-68 pA): the intersection point is in the left branch. The point can be shown to be stable.

Therefore, the ML model does not produce spikes.

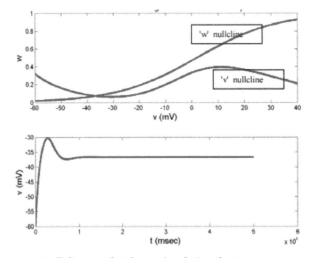

Nullclines and Voltage simulation for I = 60 pA

For I_a in the range (69-217 pA): the intersection point is in the middle branch. Therefore, the ML model produces limit cycle oscillations.

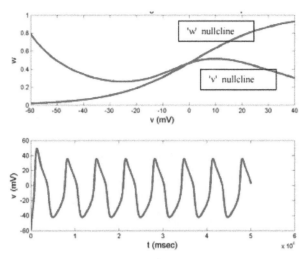

Nullclines and Voltage simulation for I = 150 pA

For I_a in the range (218 pA): the intersection point is in the right branch. Therefore, the membrane voltage exhibits depolarization.

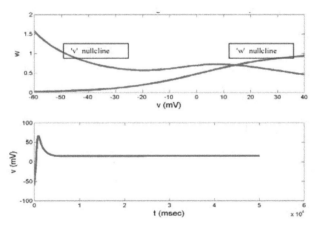

Nullclines and Voltage simulation for I = 300 pA

I_{NAPK} Model

So far we have visited two simplified neuron models that are capable of exhibiting some of the basic dynamic properties of a neuron: resting state, oscillations and depolarization. Both the models are 2-variable systems which are preferred since they can be studied conveniently using phase-plane techniques. The FitzHugh-Nagumo model was reduced systematically and derived from the HH model, whereas the Morris-Lecas model is slightly different from the HH model.

Let us now consider another model that is constructed by systematic reduction from the HH model. This reduced model, known as the Ina,p + IK model has a persistent sodium channel and a potassium channel. The "persistent" sodium channel, has only an activation variable; there is no inactivation variable. The potassium channel also has a single activation variable.

Membrane voltage dynamics of such a model can be written as usual in the following form:

$$C\frac{dv}{dt} = I_a - \bar{g}_{Na}m(v - E_{Na}) - \bar{g}_k n(v - E_k) - g_L(v - E_L)$$

$$\tau_m \frac{dm}{dt} = (-m + m_\infty)$$

$$\tau_n \frac{dn}{dt} = (-n + n_\infty)$$

If we assume that 'm' dynamics is fast, we replace m in eqn. above with m_∞ and eliminate the 'm' dynamics. We are now left with the following two equations:

$$C\frac{dv}{dt} = I_a - \bar{g}_{Na}m_\infty(v - E_{Na}) - \bar{g}_k n(v - E_k) - g_L(v - E_L)$$

$$\tau_n \frac{dn}{dt} = (-n + n_\infty)$$

$$c = 1; \bar{g}_{Na} = 20; E_{Na} = 60mV; \bar{g}_k = 10; E_k = -90mV; g_L = 8; E_L = -80mV$$

m_∞ and τ_m are modeled on the lines of eqns.

$$m_\infty = \frac{1}{1 + \exp\left[(V_{1/2} - V)/\lambda\right]}$$

$$\tau_m(V) = C_{base} + C_{amp}\exp\left[-(V_{max} - V)^2/\sigma^2\right]$$

Thus, the parameters for m_∞ are:

$V_{1/2}$ = -20 mV and λ = 15,

And the parameters for n_∞ are,

$V_{1/2}$ = -25 mV and λ = 5. $\tau_n(V) = 1$ for all V.

Rewriting eqns. (5.3.4, 5.3.5) above, we may express the V- and n- null-clines as follows:

V-nullcine:

$$n = \frac{I_a - \bar{g}_{Na}m_\infty(v - E_{Na}) - g_L(v - E_L)}{\bar{g}_k n(v - E_k)}$$

and

n-nullcline:

$$n = n_\infty(V)$$

The V- and n-nullclines obtained from the above equations are shown in fig. for I_a = 60 pA and 500 pA.

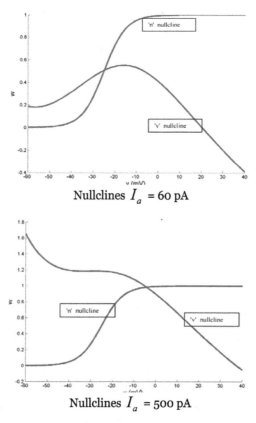

Nullclines I_a = 60 pA

Nullclines I_a = 500 pA

A Simplified two-dimensional Model

The three models visited above in this chapter have certain common features. They differ in the ion channel composition; they are derived from different cell models by different steps of simplification. But all three share certain features of dynamics. All the three models have:

- Resting state for I = 0

- Spikes/oscillations/limit cycles for a sufficiently large I.

- An N-shaped V-nullcline. The shape of the second nullcline is linear in the FN model, and sigmoidal in ML and INAPK model.

- The intersection between the V-nullcine and the second nullcline near the U- shaped, lower arch of the V-nullcline plays a crucial role in neuron dynamics.

When the second nullcline intersects the V-nullcline in the 1st branch there is a resting state; when the intersection occurs in the middle branch there are oscillations.

Consider the role of the remaining part of the state space. In the FN model for example, when the external current I = 0. When the initial voltage (V(0)) is less than 'a', the system returns to the resting potential, 0. But if V(0) > a, the neuron state (V, w) increases until it touches the 3rd branch of the V-nullcline, climbs up towards the maximum of the V-nullcline, turns leftwards at the maximum, proceeds up to the 1st branch of the V-nullcline, before it slides down the 3rd branch to the resting state. Thus the remaining part of the phase-plane determines the downstroke and the peak of the action potential.

When the intersection point shifts slightly from the left of the minimum of V- nullcline (where the system exhibits excitability) to the right of the minimum (where the system oscillates), the shape and size of the action potential are about the same. Thus in the oscillatory regime too, the part of the phase-space other than the shaded portion shown in fig. merely contributes to downstroke and the peak value of the action potential.

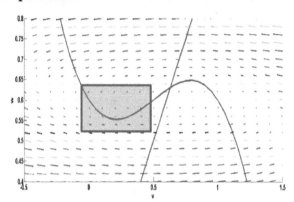

Area of interest for the upstroke: Phase plane analysis- Oscillations (FN model) at a=0.5; b = 0.1; r=0.1; I_a =0.6

Similar comments can be said about the dynamics in the other two models also.

Thus the above three systems can be reduced to a more general, simpler system as follows. The U-shaped, lower arch of the V-nullcline is approximated by a quadratic function. Since only the shape of the second null-cline at its intersection with V-nullcline matters, and not its shape elsewhere, the second nullcline is approximated by a straightline. Dynamics far from the intersection point are implemented by a simple resetting once the membrane voltage hits a peak value or a minimum.

The quadratic approximation of the V-nullcline at its minimum is given as,

$$u = u_{min} + p(V - V_{min})^2$$

The linear approximation of the second nullcline may be expressed as,

$$u = s(V - V_0)$$

The dynamics of the reduced system then becomes,

$$\tau_V \frac{dV}{dt} = -u + u_{min} + p(V - V_{min})^2$$

$$\tau_u \frac{du}{dt} = -u + s(V - V_0)$$

Where τ_V and τ_u denote the time-scales of V- and u-dynamics. Since V and u denote the fast and slow variables respectively, $\tau_V << \tau_u$.

If the V-dynamics of Eqn. above is implemented without any auxiliary conditions, V blows up to infinity in a finite time 't'. This can be shown easily on integrating Eqn. as:

$$V = c_1 * \tan(c_2 t)$$

Therefore, the downstroke of the action potential is modeled by resetting V(t) when it reaches the peak value V_{max} as follows.

$$(V, u) \leftarrow (V_{reset}, u + u_{reset}), when \ V = V_{max}$$

When the membrane voltage exceeds V_{max} both V and u are reset instantaneously as specified by the above equation.

Eqns. may be rewritten in a simpler form as,

$$\frac{dv}{dt} = I + v^2 - u$$

$$\frac{du}{dt} = a(bv - u)$$

$$If \ v \geq 1, \ v \leftarrow c, u \leftarrow u + d$$

a,b,c,d = constants;

The last set of eqns. is generally referred to as the Izhikevich neuron model in current literature. Its merit lies in the low computational cost, and the ability to reproduce firing patterns of a large variety of neurons (E.M. Izhikevich et al, 2004, 2004).

Quadratic Integrate and Fire Neuron:

There is a simpler, one-dimensional version of the Izhikevich model of eqns. This model, known as the quadratic integrate and fire neuron model (Latham et al., 2000) consists of only the membrane voltage dynamics with quadratic nonlinearity:

$$\frac{dV}{dt} = I + V^2$$

$$If \ V \geq V_{peak}, \ V \leftarrow V_{reset}$$

Note that for any non-zero value of I or V(o), eqns. above blows up in a finite time, as already shown above on Eqn. The resetting condition of eqn. prevents the blowing up.

By appropriate choice of the model parameters - c- the above model can be made to express a variety of neurodynamic behaviors.

If $I < 0$, $\dot{V} = 0$ at two values, $V = \pm\sqrt{-I}$. Let us call these roots, $V_{threshold} = \sqrt{-I}$ and $V_{rest} = \sqrt{-I}$. These names can be easily justified.

For $V > V_{threshold}$, $\dot{V} > 0$. Therefore, V increases indefinitely.

Similarly, $V_{rest} < V < V_{threshold}$, $\dot{V} > 0$ and therefore V decreases towards V_{rest}. Therefore $V = V_{threshold}$ is an unstable point.

For $V_{rest} > V$, $\dot{V} > 0$, Therefore, V increases towards V_{rest}. Hence $V = V_{rest}$ is a stable state.

Now consider the dynamics of the neurons in the following 3 cases:

Case i

For I < 0, $I < 0$, $V_{threshold} = \sqrt{-I}$ and $V_{rest} = \sqrt{-I}$ are real numbers.

If $V(0) < V_{threshold}$, V approaches V_{rest} and remain there forever.

If $V(0) > V_{threshold}$, V grows indefinitely and, unless clamped, reaches infinity in a finite time.

The reset condition of eqn. prevents the runaway of V, and resets it to V_{reset} as soon as V reaches V_{peak}.

Since $V_{reset} < V_{rest}$, V now tends to V_{rest} and settles there. This latter behavior is described as 'excitability.' It is analogous to the case of FN model when I = 0.

Excitable behavior may be produced not just by the initial condition, but also by giving a series of pulses which progressively push the membrane voltage towards $V_{threshold}$ and beyond, causing excitation.

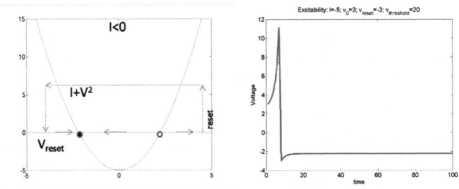

a) Reset condition b) Voltage simulation at I = 5; V_0 = 3; V_{reset} = -3; $V_{threshold}$ = 20;

Case ii:

In this case, the model behavior for $V(0) < V_{threshold}$ is similar to that of the previous case. But when $V(0) > V_{threshold}$, V quickly reaches V_{peak} and gets reset to V_{reset}. But instead of a slow return to V_{rest}, it rises again and again to V_{peak} exhibiting continuous, periodic firing. Thus the model in case (ii) exhibits two stable states: one corresponding to the resting state, and the other the state of continuous firing. The model is therefore said to have bistability.

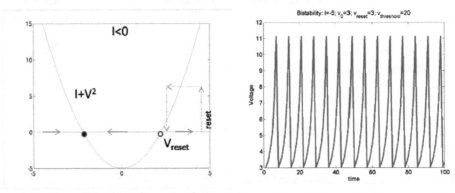

a) Reset condition b) Voltage simulation at I = -5; V_0 = 3; V_{reset} = 3; $V_{threshold}$ = 20;

Case (iii): I > 0

When I > 0 and $V_{threshold} = \sqrt{-I}$ and $V_{rest} = \sqrt{-I}$ are unreal. Therefore V rapidly approaches V_{peak} and gets reset to V_{rest} again and again.

This neuron shows tonic firing, even without excitation.

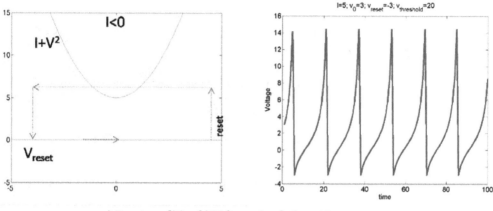

a) Reset condition b) Voltage simulation at I = 5;   = 3;

Leaky Integrate and Fire Neuron Model

This is the simplest model of spike generation. An electric circuit implementation of it consists of a capacitance charged by a current, and discharged whenever the voltage across the capacitance exceeds a limit.

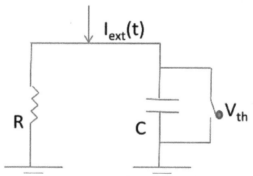

Leaky Integrate and Fire circuit diagram

Applying the Kirchoff's current law of electric circuits, the external current, I_{ext}, going into the circuit may be expressed as,

$$C\frac{dv}{dt} + \frac{V}{R} = I_{ext}(t)$$

Capacitance is discharged whenever, $V > \theta$, a threshold value. It is assumed that whenever the capacitor is charged, the "neuron" emits a spike. Note that in this model, there is no nonlinear, explosive build of excitation reaching a peak producing an action potential. The spike generated in this neuron model is more notional. This has always been one of the points of criticism about the leaky integrate and fire model.

If the capacitance starts off at o voltage, let us consider the time taken by the capacitance to reach the threshold, θ.

If I_{ext} is a constant current, I_0, voltage variation while the capacitance is charging may be expressed as,

$$V(t) = RI_0\left(1 - \exp(-t/\tau)\right)$$

where τ the time-constant of the circuit equals RC. Since the charging stops at $V=\theta$, the time taken, T, to reach this threshold is given by setting $V(t)=\theta$, or,

$$\theta = RI_0(1 - \exp(-T/\tau))$$

Or

$$T = \tau \ln\left(RI_0 / \left(RI_0 - \theta\right)\right)$$

Since there is a spike every time the capacitance discharges, spike frequency, f, is the reciprocal of T.

$$f = 1/\tau \ln\left(RI_0 / \left(RI_0 - \theta\right)\right)$$

A key property of a real neuron reproduced by the above model is thresholding effect. Note that the model exhibits firing only when $RI_0 > \theta$. But as I_0 increases beyond R/θ, f increases indefinitely, instead of saturating as it happens in a real neuron.

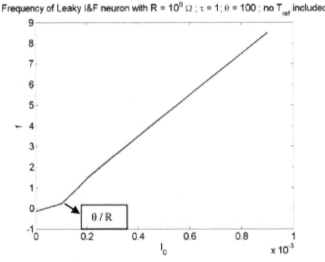

frequency vs I_0 without inclusion of absolute refractory period

In order to restore the saturation property, the condition of absolute refractory period is introduced into the above model. Accordingly the capacitance can begin to be charged only a little while, T_{ref}, after the external current is applied. Therefore, the time taken to charge is incremented as,

$$T = \tau \ln\left(RI_0 / \left(RI_0 - \theta\right)\right) + T_{ref}$$

And the new firing rate is,

$$f = \frac{1}{\tau \ln \left(RI_0 / \left(RI_0 - \theta \right) \right) + T_{ref}}$$

With the inclusion of absolute refractory period, the plot of $I_0\ vs\ f$, shows saturating behavior.

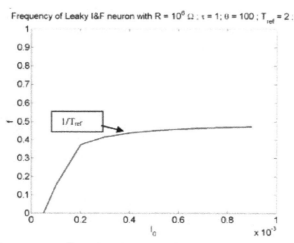

frequency vs I_0 with inclusion of absolute refractory period

Galves–Löcherbach Model

The Galves–Löcherbach model is a model with intrinsic stochasticity for biological neural nets, in which the probability of a future spike depends on the evolution of the complete system since the last spike. This model of spiking neurons was developed by mathematicians Antonio Galves and Eva Löcherbach. In the first article on the model, in 2013, they called it a model of a "system with interacting stochastic chains with memory of variable length."

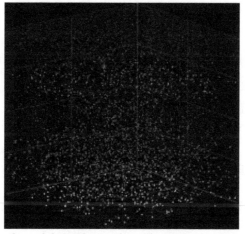

3D Vizualization of Galves–Löcherbach model simulating the spiking of 4000 neurons (4 layers with one population of inhibitory neurons and one population of excitatory neurons each) in 180 time intervals

History

Some inspirations of the Galves–Löcherbach model are the Frank Spitzer's interacting particle system and Jorma Rissanen's notion of stochastic chain with memory of variable length. Another work that influenced this model was Bruno Cessac's study on the leaky integrate-and-fire model, who himself was influenced by Hédi Soula. Galves and Löcherbach referred to the process that Cessac described as "a version in a finite dimension" of their own probabilistic model.

Prior integrate-and-fire models with stochastic characteristics relied on including a noise to simulate stochasticity. The Galves–Löcherbach model distinguishes itself because it is inherently stochastic, incorporating probabilistic measures directly in the calculation of spikes. It is also a model that may be applied relatively easily, from a computational standpoint, with a good ratio between cost and efficiency. It remains a non-Markovian model, since the probability of a given neuronal spike depends on the accumulated activity of the system since the last spike.

Contributions to the model were made, considering the hydrodynamic limit of the interacting neuronal system, the long-range behavior and aspects pertaining to the process in the sense of predicting and classifying behaviors according to a fonction of parameters, and the generalization of the model to the continuous time.

The Galves–Löcherbach model was a cornerstone to the Research, Innocation and Dissemination Center for Neuromathematics.

Formal Definition

The model considers a countable set of neurons I and models its evolution in discrete-time periods $t \in \mathbb{Z}$ with a stochastic chain $(X_t)_{t \in \mathbb{Z}}$, considering values in $\{0,1\}^I$. More precisely, for each neuron $i \in I$ and time period $t \in \mathbb{Z}$, we define $X_t(i) = 1$ if neuron i spikes in period t, and conversely $X_t(i) = 0$. The configuration of the set of neurons, in the time period $t \in \mathbb{Z}$, is therefore defined as $X_t = (X_t(i), i \in I)$. For each time period $t \in \mathbb{Z}$, we define a sigma-algebra $\mathcal{F}_t = \sigma(X_s(j), j \in I, s \leq t)$, representing the history of the evolution of the activity of this set of neurons until the relevant time period t. The dynamics of the activity of this set of neurons is defined as follows. Once the history $\mathcal{F}_{t-1}$ is given, neurons spike or not in the next time period t independently from one another, that is, for each finite subset $F \subset I$ and any configuration a $a_i \in \{0,1\}, i \in F$ we have

$$\text{Prob}(X_t(i) = a_i, i \in I \mid \mathcal{F}_{t-1}) = \prod_{i \in I} \text{Prob}(X_t(i) = a_i \mid \mathcal{F}_{t-1}).$$

Furthermore, the probability that a given neuron i spikes in a time period t, according to the probabilistic model, is described by the formula

$$\text{Prob}(X_t(i) = 1 \mid \mathcal{F}_{t-1}) = \phi_i \left(\sum_{j \in I} W_{j \to i} \sum_{s=L_t^i}^{t-1} g_j(t-s) X_s(j), t - L_t^i \right)$$

where $W_{j \to i}$ is synaptic weight that expresses the increase of membrane potential of neuron i because of neuron j's spike,   is a function that models the leak of potential and L_t^i is the most recent period of neuron i's spike before the given time period t, considering the formula

$$L_t^i = \sup\{s < t : X_s(i) = 1\}.$$

At time s before t, neuron i spikes, restoring the membrane potential to its initial value.

Binary Neuron Models

The simplified neuron models visited so far in this chapter are models of action potential or spike generation. If we wish to simply the single neuron model further, we may consider rate-coded models which represent the neuron state in terms of the spike rate. These models typically describe neurons as binary elements, with a high (excited state) and a low (resting) state.

Dynamic Binary Neuron Model

A dynamic version of a binary neuron is a bistableneuron whose dynamics is described as,

$$\tau\dot{u} = -u + V + I$$
$$V = \tanh(\lambda u)$$

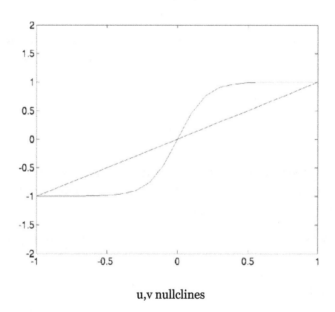

u,v nullclines

V is an abstract quantity that denotes if the neuron is excited (V is close to 1) or in the resting state (V is close to -1).

For I = 0 and $\lambda>1$, the above system has three fixed points. The fixed point at the origin can be shown to be unstable, while the ones on the flanks can be shown to be stable. When released from a random initial condition, the neuron state, V, settles near +1 or -1.

For I > b, where b = 2.63, and $\lambda>1$, Eqn above has only a single, stable fixed point at V close to +1.

For I < -b, and $\lambda>1$, eqn above has only a single, stable fixed point at V close to -1.

For −b < I < b, there are again three fixed points, two close to + 1 and -1 respectively, and the third somewhere in the middle, not necessarily at the origin.

The above neuron model also shows hysteresis effect. If I is reduced from a large positive value to a large negative value and back, the points at which V makes transitions from (+1 to -1 and vice versa) are different in the forward pass and the reverse pass.

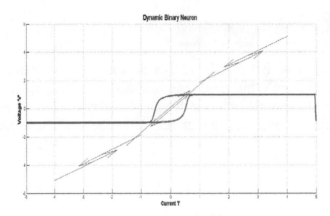

Hysteresis curve for a dynamic binary neuron

Static Binary Neuron Model

The McCulloch and Pitts neuron model is a good example of a static binary neuron. It combines the inputs, xi, that it receives from other neurons and computes its output, y. The relationship between the inputs xi and the output y is given as,

$$y = g\left(\sum_{i=1}^{n} w_i x_i - \theta\right)$$

Where wi s are the synaptic strengths, or the "weights" of the connections from the neurons that send inputs to the neuron of interest; q is the threshold for excitation; g(.) is known as a transfer function, which typically has a sigmoidal shape.

Four types of transfer functions are usually considered depending on the range of values that y is permitted.

Hardlimiting nonlinearity:

y = 1/0:

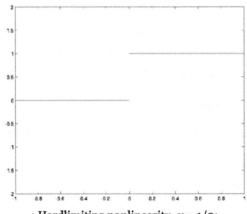

: Hardlimiting nonlinearity- y = 1/0:

y = +1.

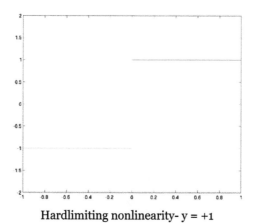

Hardlimiting nonlinearity- y = +1

Smooth sigmoid nonlinearity:

Logistic function:

$$y \in (0,1)$$

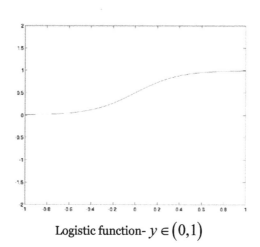

Logistic function- $y \in (0,1)$

Tanh(.) function:

$$y \in (-1,1)$$

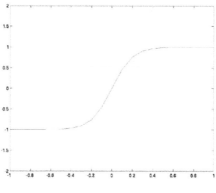

Tanh(.) function - $y \in (-1,1)$

References

- Tsumoto, Kunichika; Kitajimab, Hiroyuki; Yoshinagac, Tetsuya; Aiharad, Kazuyuki; Kawakamif, Hiroshi (January 2006), "Bifurcations in Morris–Lecar neuron model" (PDF), Neurocomputing (in English and Japanese), 69 (4–6): 293–316, doi:10.1016/j.neucom.2005.03.006

- B. Cessac, "A discrete time neural network model with spiking neurons: II: Dynamics with noise". Journal of Mathematical Biology, Vol. 62, n° 6, pg 863–900. Jun. 2011

- F. C. Hoppensteadt and E. M. Izhikevich (1997). Weakly connected neural networks. Springer. p. 4. ISBN 978-0-387-94948-2

- Potluri, Pushpa Sree (26 November 2014). "Error Correction Capacity of Unary Coding". Retrieved 10 March 2017

- Morris, Catherine; Lecar, Harold (July 1981), "Voltage Oscillations in the barnacle giant muscle fiber", Biophys J., 35 (1): 193–213, doi:10.1016/S0006-3495(81)84782-0, PMC 1327511 , PMID 7260316

- A. De Masi, A. Galves, E. Löcherbach, E. Presutti, "Hydrodynamic limit for interacting neurons". Journal of Statistical Physics, 158(4), 866–902, 2015

- Martin Anthony (January 2001). Discrete Mathematics of Neural Networks: Selected Topics. SIAM. pp. 3–. ISBN 978-0-89871-480-7

- Maan, A. K.; Jayadevi, D. A.; James, A. P. (1 January 2016). "A Survey of Memristive Threshold Logic Circuits". IEEE Transactions on Neural Networks and Learning Systems. PP (99): 1–13. doi:10.1109/TNNLS.2016.2547842. ISSN 2162-237X

- Keynes, RD; Rojas, E; Taylor, RE; Vergara, J (March 1973), "Calcium and potassium systems of a giant barnacle muscle fibre under membrane potential control", The Journal of Physiology (London), 229: 409–455, PMC 1350315 , PMID 4724831

- Charu C. Aggarwal (25 July 2014). Data Classification: Algorithms and Applications. CRC Press. pp. 209–. ISBN 978-1-4665-8674-1

- Paul Werbos, Backpropagation through time: what it does and how to do it. Proceedings of the IEEE, Volume 78, Issue 10, 1550–1560, Oct 1990, doi10.1109/5.58337

An Overview of Artificial Neural Networks

Artificial neural networks are made up of connected artificial neurons, which carry activation signals. One of the most prominent types of artificial neural network is recurrent neural network. The connection formed through this are in a directed cycle form. The major components of neural networks are discussed in this chapter.

Artificial Neural Network

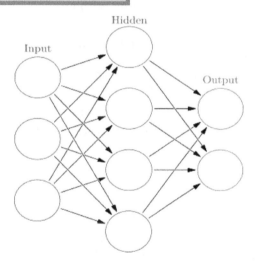

An artificial neural network is an interconnected group of nodes, akin to the vast network of neurons in a brain. Here, each circular node represents an artificial neuron and an arrow represents a connection from the output of one neuron to the input of another.

Artificial neural networks (ANNs) or connectionist systems are a computational model used in machine learning, computer science and other research disciplines, which is based on a large collection of connected simple units called artificial neurons, loosely analogous to axons in a biological brain. Connections between neurons carry an activation signal of varying strength. If the combined incoming signals are strong enough, the neuron becomes activated and the signal travels to other neurons connected to it. Such systems can be trained from examples, rather than explicitly programmed, and excel in areas where the solution or feature detection is difficult to express in a traditional computer program. Like other machine learning methods, neural networks have been used to solve a wide variety of tasks, like computer vision and speech recognition, that are difficult to solve using ordinary rule-based programming.

Typically, neurons are connected in layers, and signals travel from the first (input), to the last (output) layer. Modern neural network projects typically have a few thousand to a few million neural units and millions of connections; their computing power is similar to a worm brain, several orders of magnitude simpler than a human brain. The signals and state of artificial neurons are real numbers, typically between 0 and 1. There may be a threshold function or limiting function on each connection and on the unit itself, such that the signal must surpass the limit before propagating. Back propagation is the use of forward stimulation to modify connection weights, and is sometimes done to train the network using known correct outputs. However, the success is unpredictable: after training, some systems are good at solving problems while others are not. Training typically requires several thousand cycles of interaction.

The goal of the neural network is to solve problems in the same way that a human would, although several neural network categories are more abstract. New brain research often stimulates new patterns in neural networks. One new approach is use of connections which span further to connect processing layers rather than adjacent neurons. Other research being explored with the different types of signal over time that axons propagate, such as deep learning, interpolates greater complexity than a set of boolean variables being simply on or off. Newer types of network are more free flowing in terms of stimulation and inhibition, with connections interacting in more chaotic and complex ways. Dynamic neural networks are the most advanced, in that they dynamically can, based on rules, form new connections and even new neural units while disabling others.

Historically, the use of neural network models marked a directional shift in the late 1980s from high-level (symbolic) artificial intelligence, characterized by expert systems with knowledge embodied in *if-then* rules, to low-level (sub-symbolic) machine learning, characterized by knowledge embodied in the parameters of a cognitive model with some dynamical system.

History

Warren McCulloch and Walter Pitts (1943) created a computational model for neural networks based on mathematics and algorithms called threshold logic. This model paved the way for neural network research to split into two distinct approaches. One approach focused on biological processes in the brain and the other focused on the application of neural networks to artificial intelligence. This work led to the influential paper by Kleene on nerve networks and their link to finite automata.

1. "Representation of events in nerve nets and finite automata." In: Automata Studies, ed. by C.E. Shannon and J. McCarthy. Annals of Mathematics Studies, no. 34. Princeton University Press, Princeton, N. J.

Hebbian Learning

In the late 1940s psychologist Donald Hebb created a hypothesis of learning based on the mechanism of neural plasticity that is now known as Hebbian learning. Hebbian learning is considered to be a 'typical' unsupervised learning rule and its later variants were early models for long term potentiation. Researchers started applying these ideas to computational models in 1948 with Turing's B-type machines.

Farley and Wesley A. Clark (1954) first used computational machines, then called "calculators", to simulate a Hebbian network at MIT. Other neural network computational machines were created by Rochester, Holland, Habit, and Duda (1956).

Frank Rosenblatt (1958) created the perceptron, an algorithm for pattern recognition based on a two-layer computer learning network using simple addition and subtraction. With mathematical notation, Rosenblatt also described circuitry not in the basic perceptron, such as the exclusive-or circuit, a circuit which could not be processed by neural networks until after the backpropagation algorithm was created by Paul Werbos (1975).

Neural network research stagnated after the publication of machine learning research by Marvin Minsky and Seymour Papert (1969), who discovered two key issues with the computational machines that processed neural networks. The first was that basic perceptrons were incapable of processing the exclusive-or circuit. The second significant issue was that computers didn't have enough processing power to effectively handle the long run time required by large neural networks. Neural network research slowed until computers achieved greater processing power.

Backpropagation and Resurgence

A key advance that came later was the backpropagation algorithm which effectively solved the exclusive-or problem, and more generally the problem of quickly training multi-layer neural networks (Werbos 1975).

In the mid-1980s, parallel distributed processing became popular under the name connectionism. The textbook by David E. Rumelhart and James McClelland (1986) provided a full exposition of the use of connectionism in computers to simulate neural processes.

Neural networks, as used in artificial intelligence, have traditionally been viewed as simplified models of neural processing in the brain, even though the relation between this model and the biological architecture of the brain is debated; it's not clear to what degree artificial neural networks mirror brain function.

Support vector machines and other, much simpler methods such as linear classifiers gradually overtook neural networks in machine learning popularity. As earlier challenges in training deep neural networks were successfully addressed with methods such as Unsupervised Pre-training and computing power increased through the use of GPUs and distributed computing, neural networks were again deployed on a large scale, particularly in image and visual recognition problems. This became known as "deep learning", although deep learning is not strictly synonymous with deep neural networks.

Improvements Since 2006

Computational devices have been created in CMOS, for both biophysical simulation and neuromorphic computing. More recent efforts show promise for creating nanodevices for very large scale principal components analyses and convolution. If successful, it would create a new class of neural computing because it depends on learning rather than programming and because it is fundamentally analog rather than digital even though the first instantiations may in fact be with CMOS digital devices.

Between 2009 and 2012, the recurrent neural networks and deep feedforward neural networks developed in the research group of Jürgen Schmidhuber at the Swiss AI Lab IDSIA have won eight international competitions in pattern recognition and machine learning. For example, the bi-directional and multi-dimensional long short-term memory (LSTM) of Alex Graves et al. won three competitions in connected handwriting recognition at the 2009 International Conference on Document Analysis and Recognition (ICDAR), without any prior knowledge about the three different languages to be learned.

Fast GPU-based implementations of this approach by Dan Ciresan and colleagues at IDSIA have won several pattern recognition contests, including the IJCNN 2011 Traffic Sign Recognition Competition, the ISBI 2012 Segmentation of Neuronal Structures in Electron Microscopy Stacks challenge, and others. Their neural networks also were the first artificial pattern recognizers to achieve human-competitive or even superhuman performance on important benchmarks such as traffic sign recognition (IJCNN 2012), or the MNIST handwritten digits problem of Yann LeCun at NYU.

Deep, highly nonlinear neural architectures similar to the 1980 neocognitron by Kunihiko Fukushima and the "standard architecture of vision", inspired by the simple and complex cells identified by David H. Hubel and Torsten Wiesel in the primary visual cortex, can also be pre-trained by unsupervised methods of Geoff Hinton's lab at University of Toronto. A team from this lab won a 2012 contest sponsored by Merck to design software to help find molecules that might lead to new drugs.

Models

Neural network models in artificial intelligence are usually referred to as artificial neural networks (ANNs); these are essentially simple mathematical models defining a function $f : X \rightarrow Y$ or a distribution over X or both X and Y, but sometimes models are also intimately associated with a particular learning algorithm or learning rule. A common use of the phrase "ANN model" is really the definition of a *class* of such functions (where members of the class are obtained by varying parameters, connection weights, or specifics of the architecture such as the number of neurons or their connectivity).

Network Function

The word *network* in the term 'artificial neural network' refers to the interconnections between the neurons in the different layers of each system. An example system has three layers. The first layer has input neurons which send data via synapses to the second layer of neurons, and then via more synapses to the third layer of output neurons. More complex systems will have more layers of neurons, some having increased layers of input neurons and output neurons. The synapses store parameters called "weights" that manipulate the data in the calculations.

An ANN is typically defined by three types of parameters:

1. The interconnection pattern between the different layers of neurons

2. The weights of the interconnections, which are updated in the learning process.

3. The activation function that converts a neuron's weighted input to its output activation.

Mathematically, a neuron's network function $f(x)$ is defined as a composition of other functions $g_i(x)$, which can further be defined as a composition of other functions. This can be conveniently represented as a network structure, with arrows depicting the dependencies between variables.

A widely used type of composition is the *nonlinear weighted sum*, where $f(x) = K\left(\sum_i w_i g_i(x)\right)$,

where K (commonly referred to as the activation function) is some predefined function, such as the hyperbolic tangent or sigmoid function. The important characteristic of the activation function is that it provides a smooth transition as input values change, i.e. a small change in input produces a small change in output. It will be convenient for the following to refer to a collection of functions g_i as simply a vector $g = (g_1, g_2, \ldots, g_n)$.

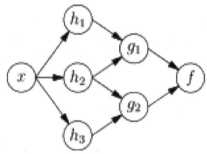

ANN dependency graph

This figure depicts such a decomposition of f, with dependencies between variables indicated by arrows. These can be interpreted in two ways.

The first view is the functional view: the input x is transformed into a 3-dimensional vector h, which is then transformed into a 2-dimensional vector g, which is finally transformed into f. This view is most commonly encountered in the context of optimization.

The second view is the probabilistic view: the random variable $F = f(G)$ depends upon the random variable $G = g(H)$, which depends upon $H = h(X)$, which depends upon the random variable X. This view is most commonly encountered in the context of graphical models.

The two views are largely equivalent. In either case, for this particular network architecture, the components of individual layers are independent of each other (e.g., the components of g are independent of each other given their input h). This naturally enables a degree of parallelism in the implementation.

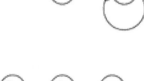

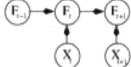

Two separate depictions of the recurrent ANN dependency graph

Networks such as the previous one are commonly called feedforward, because their graph is a directed acyclic graph. Networks with cycles are commonly called recurrent. Such networks are commonly depicted in the manner shown at the top of the figure, where f is shown as being dependent upon itself. However, an implied temporal dependence is not shown.

Learning

What has attracted the most interest in neural networks is the possibility of *learning*. Given a specific *task* to solve, and a *class* of functions F, learning means using a set of *observations* to find $f^* \in F$ which solves the task in some *optimal* sense.

This entails defining a cost function $C : F \to \mathbb{R}$ such that, for the optimal solution f^*, $C(f^*) \le C(f)$ $\forall f \in F$ – i.e., no solution has a cost less than the cost of the optimal solution.

The cost function C is an important concept in learning, as it is a measure of how far away a particular solution is from an optimal solution to the problem to be solved. Learning algorithms search through the solution space to find a function that has the smallest possible cost.

For applications where the solution is dependent on some data, the cost must necessarily be a *function of the observations*, otherwise we would not be modelling anything related to the data. It is frequently defined as a statistic to which only approximations can be made. As a simple example, consider the problem of finding the model f, which minimizes $C = E\left[(f(x) - y)^2 \right]$, for data pairs (x, y) drawn from some distribution $\mathcal{D}$. In practical situations we would only have N samples from $\mathcal{D}$ and thus, for the above example, we would only minimize $\hat{C} = \frac{1}{N} \sum_{i=1}^{N} (f(x_i) - y_i)^2$. Thus, the cost is minimized over a sample of the data rather than the entire distribution generating the data.

When $N \to \infty$ some form of online machine learning must be used, where the cost is partially minimized as each new example is seen. While online machine learning is often used when $\mathcal{D}$ is fixed, it is most useful in the case where the distribution changes slowly over time. In neural network methods, some form of online machine learning is frequently used for finite datasets.

Choosing a Cost Function

While it is possible to define some arbitrary ad hoc cost function, frequently a particular cost will be used, either because it has desirable properties (such as convexity) or because it arises naturally from a particular formulation of the problem (e.g., in a probabilistic formulation the posterior probability of the model can be used as an inverse cost). Ultimately, the cost function will depend on the desired task. An overview of the three main categories of learning tasks is provided below:

Learning Paradigms

There are three major learning paradigms, each corresponding to a particular abstract learning task. These are supervised learning, unsupervised learning and reinforcement learning.

Supervised Learning

In supervised learning, we are given a set of example pairs $(x, y), x \in X, y \in Y$ and the aim is to find a function $f : X \to Y$ in the allowed class of functions that matches the examples. In other words, we wish to *infer* the mapping implied by the data; the cost function is related to the mismatch between our mapping and the data and it implicitly contains prior knowledge about the problem domain.

A commonly used cost is the mean-squared error, which tries to minimize the average squared error between the network's output, $f(x)$, and the target value y over all the example pairs. When one tries to minimize this cost using gradient descent for the class of neural networks called multilayer perceptrons (MLP), one obtains the common and well-known backpropagation algorithm for training neural networks.

Tasks that fall within the paradigm of supervised learning are pattern recognition (also known as classification) and regression (also known as function approximation). The supervised learning paradigm is also applicable to sequential data (e.g., for speech and gesture recognition). This can be thought of as learning with a "teacher", in the form of a function that provides continuous feedback on the quality of solutions obtained thus far.

Unsupervised Learning

In unsupervised learning, some data x is given and the cost function to be minimized, that can be any function of the data x and the network's output, f.

The cost function is dependent on the task (what we are trying to model) and our *a priori* assumptions (the implicit properties of our model, its parameters and the observed variables).

As a trivial example, consider the model $f(x) = a$ where a is a constant and the cost $C = E[(x - f(x))^2]$. Minimizing this cost will give us a value of a that is equal to the mean of the data. The cost function can be much more complicated. Its form depends on the application: for example, in compression it could be related to the mutual information between x and $f(x)$, whereas in statistical modeling, it could be related to the posterior probability of the model given the data (note that in both of those examples those quantities would be maximized rather than minimized).

Tasks that fall within the paradigm of unsupervised learning are in general estimation problems; the applications include clustering, the estimation of statistical distributions, compression and filtering.

Reinforcement Learning

In reinforcement learning, data x are usually not given, but generated by an agent's interactions with the environment. At each point in time t, the agent performs an action y_t and the environment generates an observation x_t and an instantaneous cost c_t, according to some (usually unknown) dynamics. The aim is to discover a *policy* for selecting actions that minimizes some measure of a long-term cost, e.g., the expected cumulative cost. The environment's dynamics and the long-term cost for each policy are usually unknown, but can be estimated.

More formally the environment is modeled as a Markov decision process (MDP) with states $s_1, ..., s_n \in S$ and actions $a_1, ..., a_m \in A$ with the following probability distributions: the instantaneous cost distribution $P(c_t \mid s_t)$, the observation distribution $P(x_t \mid s_t)$ and the transition $P(s_{t+1} \mid s_t, a_t)$, while a policy is defined as the conditional distribution over actions given the observations. Taken together, the two then define a Markov chain (MC). The aim is to discover the policy (i.e., the MC) that minimizes the cost.

ANNs are frequently used in reinforcement learning as part of the overall algorithm. Dynamic programming has been coupled with ANNs (giving neurodynamic programming) by Bertsekas and Tsitsiklis and applied to multi-dimensional nonlinear problems such as those involved in vehicle routing, natural resources management or medicine because of the ability of ANNs to mitigate losses of accuracy even when reducing the discretization grid density for numerically approximating the solution of the original control problems.

Tasks that fall within the paradigm of reinforcement learning are control problems, games and other sequential decision making tasks.

Learning Algorithms

Training a neural network model essentially means selecting one model from the set of allowed models (or, in a Bayesian framework, determining a distribution over the set of allowed models) that minimizes the cost criterion. There are numerous algorithms available for training neural network models; most of them can be viewed as a straightforward application of optimization theory and statistical estimation.

Most of the algorithms used in training artificial neural networks employ some form of gradient descent, using backpropagation to compute the actual gradients. This is done by simply taking the derivative of the cost function with respect to the network parameters and then changing those parameters in a gradient-related direction. The backpropagation training algorithms are usually classified into three categories:

1. steepest descent (with variable learning rate and momentum, resilient backpropagation);

2. quasi-Newton (Broyden-Fletcher-Goldfarb-Shanno, one step secant);

3. Levenberg-Marquardt and conjugate gradient (Fletcher-Reeves update, Polak-Ribiére update, Powell-Beale restart, scaled conjugate gradient).

Evolutionary methods, gene expression programming, simulated annealing, expectation-maximization, non-parametric methods and particle swarm optimization are some other methods for training neural networks.

Use

Perhaps the greatest advantage of ANNs is their ability to be used as an arbitrary function approximation mechanism that 'learns' from observed data. However, using them is not so straightforward, and a relatively good understanding of the underlying theory is essential.

- Choice of model: This will depend on the data representation and the application. Overly complex models tend to lead to challenges in learning.

- Learning algorithm: There are numerous trade-offs between learning algorithms. Almost any algorithm will work well with the *correct hyperparameters* for training on a particular fixed data set. However, selecting and tuning an algorithm for training on unseen data require a significant amount of experimentation.

- Robustness: If the model, cost function and learning algorithm are selected appropriately, the resulting ANN can be extremely robust.

With the correct implementation, ANNs can be used naturally in online learning and large data set applications. Their simple implementation and the existence of mostly local dependencies exhibited in the structure allows for fast, parallel implementations in hardware.

Applications

The utility of artificial neural network models lies in the fact that they can be used to infer a function from observations. This is particularly useful in applications where the complexity of the data or task makes the design of such a function by hand impracticable.

Real-life Applications

The tasks artificial neural networks are applied to tend to fall within the following broad categories:

- Function approximation, or regression analysis, including time series prediction, fitness approximation and modeling.

- Classification, including pattern and sequence recognition, novelty detection and sequential decision making.

- Data processing, including filtering, clustering, blind source separation and compression.

- Robotics, including directing manipulators, prosthesis.

- Control, including computer numerical control.

Application areas include the system identification and control (vehicle control, trajectory prediction, process control, natural resources management), quantum chemistry, game-playing and decision making (backgammon, chess, poker), pattern recognition (radar systems, face identification, object recognition and more), sequence recognition (gesture, speech, handwritten text recognition), medical diagnosis, financial applications (e.g. automated trading systems), data mining (or knowledge discovery in databases, "KDD"), visualization and e-mail spam filtering.

Artificial neural networks have also been used to diagnose several cancers. An ANN based hybrid lung cancer detection system named HLND improves the accuracy of diagnosis and the speed of lung cancer radiology. These networks have also been used to diagnose prostate cancer. The diagnoses can be used to make specific models taken from a large group of patients compared to information of one given patient. The models do not depend on assumptions about correlations of different variables. Colorectal cancer has also been predicted using the neural networks. Neural networks could predict the outcome for a patient with colorectal cancer with more accuracy than the current clinical methods. After training, the networks could predict multiple patient outcomes from unrelated institutions. ANN have been used to distinguish between high invasive cancer cell lines from low invasive lines using only cell shape information with almost perfect accuracy.

Neural Networks and Neuroscience

Theoretical and computational neuroscience is the field concerned with the theoretical analysis and the computational modeling of biological neural systems. Since neural systems are intimately related to cognitive processes and behavior, the field is closely related to cognitive and behavioral modeling.

The aim of the field is to create models of biological neural systems in order to understand how biological systems work. To gain this understanding, neuroscientists strive to make a link between observed biological processes (data), biologically plausible mechanisms for neural processing and learning (biological neural network models) and theory (statistical learning theory and information theory).

Types of Models

Many models are used in the field, defined at different levels of abstraction and modeling different aspects of neural systems. They range from models of the short-term behavior of individual neurons (e.g.), models of how the dynamics of neural circuitry arise from interactions between individual neurons and finally to models of how behavior can arise from abstract neural modules that represent complete subsystems. These include models of the long-term, and short-term plasticity, of neural systems and their relations to learning and memory from the individual neuron to the system level.

Networks with Memory

Integrating external memory components with artificial neural networks has a long history dating back to early research in distributed representations and self-organizing maps. E.g. in sparse distributed memory the patterns encoded by neural networks are used as memory addresses for content-addressable memory, with "neurons" essentially serving as address encoders and decoders.

More recently deep learning was shown to be useful in semantic hashing where a deep graphical model of the word-count vectors is obtained from a large set of documents. Documents are mapped to memory addresses in such a way that semantically similar documents are located at nearby addresses. Documents similar to a query document can then be found by simply accessing all the addresses that differ by only a few bits from the address of the query document.

Memory Networks is another extension to neural networks incorporating long-term memory which was developed by Facebook research. The long-term memory can be read and written to, with the goal of using it for prediction. These models have been applied in the context of question answering (QA) where the long-term memory effectively acts as a (dynamic) knowledge base, and the output is a textual response.

Neural Turing Machines developed by Google DeepMind extend the capabilities of deep neural networks by coupling them to external memory resources, which they can interact with by attentional processes. The combined system is analogous to a Turing Machine but is differentiable end-to-end, allowing it to be efficiently trained with gradient descent. Preliminary results demonstrate that Neural Turing Machines can infer simple algorithms such as copying, sorting, and associative recall from input and output examples.

Differentiable neural computers (DNC) are an extension of Neural Turing Machines, also from DeepMind. They have out-performed Neural turing machines, Long short-term memory systems and memory networks on sequence-processing tasks.

Software

Neural network software is used to simulate, research, develop and apply artificial neural networks, biological neural networks and, in some cases, a wider array of adaptive systems.

Types

Artificial neural network types vary from those with only one or two layers of single direction logic, to complicated multi–input many directional feedback loops and layers. On the whole, these systems use algorithms in their programming to determine control and organization of their functions. Most systems use "weights" to change the parameters of the throughput and the varying connections to the neurons. Artificial neural networks can be autonomous and learn by input from outside "teachers" or even self-teaching from written-in rules. Neural Cube style neural networks first pioneered by Gianna Giavelli provide a dynamic space in which networks dynamically recombine information and links across billions of self adapting nodes utilizing Neural Darwinism, a technique developed by Gerald Edelman which allows for more biologically modeled systems.

Theoretical Properties

Computational Power

The multilayer perceptron is a universal function approximator, as proven by the universal approximation theorem. However, the proof is not constructive regarding the number of neurons required, the network topology, the settings of the weights and the learning parameters.

Work by Hava Siegelmann and Eduardo D. Sontag has provided a proof that a specific recurrent architecture with rational valued weights (as opposed to full precision real number-valued weights) has the full power of a Universal Turing Machine using a finite number of neurons and standard linear connections. Further, it has been shown that the use of irrational values for weights results in a machine with super-Turing power.

Capacity

Artificial neural network models have a property called 'capacity', which roughly corresponds to their ability to model any given function. It is related to the amount of information that can be stored in the network and to the notion of complexity.

Convergence

Nothing can be said in general about convergence since it depends on a number of factors. Firstly, there may exist many local minima. This depends on the cost function and the model. Secondly, the optimization method used might not be guaranteed to converge when far away from a local minimum. Thirdly, for a very large amount of data or parameters, some methods become impractical.

In general, it has been found that theoretical guarantees regarding convergence are an unreliable guide to practical application.

Generalization and Statistics

In applications where the goal is to create a system that generalizes well in unseen examples, the problem of over-training has emerged. This arises in convoluted or over-specified systems when the capacity of the network significantly exceeds the needed free parameters. There are two schools of thought for avoiding this problem: The first is to use cross-validation and similar techniques to check for the presence of overtraining and optimally select hyperparameters such as to minimize the generalization error. The second is to use some form of *regularization*. This is a concept that emerges naturally in a probabilistic (Bayesian) framework, where the regularization can be performed by selecting a larger prior probability over simpler models; but also in statistical learning theory, where the goal is to minimize over two quantities: the 'empirical risk' and the 'structural risk', which roughly corresponds to the error over the training set and the predicted error in unseen data due to overfitting.

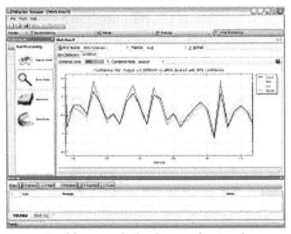

Confidence analysis of a neural network

Supervised neural networks that use a mean squared error (MSE) cost function can use formal statistical methods to determine the confidence of the trained model. The MSE on a validation set can be used as an estimate for variance. This value can then be used to calculate the confidence interval of the output of the network, assuming a normal distribution. A confidence analysis made this way is statistically valid as long as the output probability distribution stays the same and the network is not modified.

By assigning a softmax activation function, a generalization of the logistic function, on the output layer of the neural network (or a softmax component in a component-based neural network) for categorical target variables, the outputs can be interpreted as posterior probabilities. This is very useful in classification as it gives a certainty measure on classifications.

The softmax activation function is:

$$y_i = \frac{e^{x_i}}{\sum_{j=1}^{c} e^{x_j}}$$

Criticism

Training Issues

A common criticism of neural networks, particularly in robotics, is that they require a large diversity of training for real-world operation. This is not surprising, since any learning machine needs sufficient representative examples in order to capture the underlying structure that allows it to generalize to new cases. Dean A. Pomerleau, in his research presented in the paper "Knowledge-based Training of Artificial Neural Networks for Autonomous Robot Driving", uses a neural network to train a robotic vehicle to drive on multiple types of roads (single lane, multi-lane, dirt, etc.). A large amount of his research is devoted to (1) extrapolating multiple training scenarios from a single training experience, and (2) preserving past training diversity so that the system does not become overtrained (if, for example, it is presented with a series of right turns – it should not learn to always turn right). These issues are common in neural networks that must decide from amongst a wide variety of responses, but can be dealt with in several ways, for example by randomly shuffling the training examples, by using a numerical optimization algorithm that does not take too large steps when changing the network connections following an example, or by grouping examples in so-called mini-batches.

Theoretical Issues

A. K. Dewdney, a mathematician and computer scientist at University of Western Ontario and former *Scientific American* columnist, wrote in 1997, "Although neural nets do solve a few toy problems, their powers of computation are so limited that I am surprised anyone takes them seriously as a general problem-solving tool". No neural network has ever been shown that solves computationally difficult problems such as the n-Queens problem, the travelling salesman problem, or the problem of factoring large integers.

Aside from their utility, a fundamental objection to artificial neural networks is that they fail to reflect how real neurons function. Back propagation is at the heart of most artificial neural networks and not only is there no evidence of any such mechanism in natural neural networks, it seems to contradict the fundamental principle of real neurons that information can only flow forward along the axon. How information is coded by real neurons is not yet known. What is known is that sensor neurons fire action potentials more frequently with sensor activation and muscle cells pull more strongly when their associated motor neurons receive action potentials more frequently. Other than the simplest case of just relaying information from a sensor neuron to a motor neuron almost nothing of the underlying general principles of how information is handled by real neural networks is known.

The motivation behind artificial neural networks is not necessarily to replicate real neural function but to use natural neural networks as an inspiration for an approach to computing that is inherently parallel and which provides solutions to problems that have up until now been considered intractable. A central claim of artificial neural networks is therefore that it embodies some new and powerful general principle for processing information. Unfortunately, these general principles are ill-defined and it is often claimed that they are *emergent* from the neural network itself. This allows simple statistical association (the basic function of artificial neural networks) to be described as *learning* or *recognition*. As a result, artificial neural networks have a "something-for-nothing quality, one that imparts a peculiar aura of laziness and a distinct lack of curiosity about just how good these computing systems are. No human hand (or mind) intervenes; solutions are found as if by magic; and no one, it seems, has learned anything".

Hardware Issues

To implement large and effective software neural networks, considerable processing and storage resources need to be committed. While the brain has hardware tailored to the task of processing signals through a graph of neurons, simulating even a most simplified form on von Neumann architecture may compel a neural network designer to fill many millions of database rows for its connections – which can consume vast amounts of computer memory and hard disk space. Furthermore, the designer of neural network systems will often need to simulate the transmission of signals through many of these connections and their associated neurons – which must often be matched with incredible amounts of CPU processing power and time.

Jürgen Schmidhuber notes that the resurgence of neural networks in the twenty-first century, and their renewed success at image recognition tasks is largely attributable to advances in hardware: from 1991 to 2015, computing power, especially as delivered by GPGPUs (on GPUs), has increased around a million-fold, making the standard backpropagation algorithm feasible for training networks that are several layers deeper than before (but adds that this doesn't overcome algorithmic problems such as vanishing gradients "in a fundamental way"). The use of GPUs instead of ordinary CPUs can bring training times for some networks down from months to mere days.

Computing power continues to grow roughly according to Moore's Law, which may provide sufficient resources to accomplish new tasks. Neuromorphic engineering addresses the hardware difficulty directly, by constructing non-von-Neumann chips with circuits designed to implement neural nets from the ground up. Google has also designed a chip optimized for neural network processing called a Tensor Processing Unit, or TPU.

Practical Counter Examples to Criticisms

Arguments against Dewdney's position are that neural networks have been successfully used to solve many complex and diverse tasks, ranging from autonomously flying aircraft to detecting credit card fraud.

Technology writer Roger Bridgman commented on Dewdney's statements about neural nets:

Neural networks, for instance, are in the dock not only because they have been hyped to high heaven, (what hasn't?) but also because you could create a successful net without understanding how it worked: the bunch of numbers that captures its behaviour would in all probability be "an opaque, unreadable table...valueless as a scientific resource".

In spite of his emphatic declaration that science is not technology, Dewdney seems here to pillory neural nets as bad science when most of those devising them are just trying to be good engineers. An unreadable table that a useful machine could read would still be well worth having.

Although it is true that analyzing what has been learned by an artificial neural network is difficult, it is much easier to do so than to analyze what has been learned by a biological neural network.

Furthermore, researchers involved in exploring learning algorithms for neural networks are gradually uncovering generic principles which allow a learning machine to be successful. For example, Bengio and LeCun (2007) wrote an article regarding local vs non-local learning, as well as shallow vs deep architecture.

Hybrid Approaches

Some other criticisms come from advocates of hybrid models (combining neural networks and symbolic approaches), who believe that the intermix of these two approaches can better capture the mechanisms of the human mind.

Types

- Dynamic Neural Network
  - Feedforward neural network (FNN)
  - Recurrent neural network (RNN)
    - Hopfield network
    - Boltzmann machine
    - Simple recurrent networks
    - Echo state network
    - Long short-term memory
    - Bi-directional RNN
    - Hierarchical RNN
    - Stochastic neural networks
  - Kohonen Self-Organizing Maps
  - Autoencoder
  - Probabilistic neural network (PNN)
  - Time delay neural network (TDNN)
  - Regulatory feedback network (RFNN)
- Static Neural Network
  - Neocognitron
  - McCulloch-Pitts cell
  - Radial basis function network (RBF)

- o   Learning vector quantization
- o   Perceptron
    - Adaline model
    - Convolutional neural network (CNN)
- o   Modular neural networks
    - Committee of machines (COM)
    - Associative neural network (ASNN)
- Memory Network
    - o   Goog•le / Deep Mind
    - o   facebook / MemNN
    - o   Holographic associative memory
    - o   One-shot associative memory
    - o   Neural Turing Machine
    - o   Adaptive resonance theory
    - o   Hierarchical temporal memory
- Other types of networks
    - o   Instantaneously trained neural networks (ITNN)
    - o   Spiking neural network (SNN)
        - Pulse Coded Neural Networks (PCNN)
    - o   Cascading neural networks
    - o   Neuro-fuzzy networks
    - o   Growing Neural Gas (GNG)
    - o   Compositional pattern-producing networks
    - o   Counterpropagation network
    - o   Oscillating neural network
    - o   Hybridization neural network
    - o   Physical neural network
        - Optical neural network

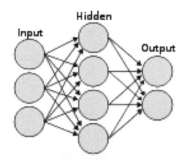

An artificial neural network.

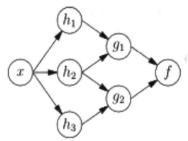

An ANN dependency graph.

Generative Adversarial Networks

Generative adversarial networks are a type of artificial intelligence algorithms used in unsupervised machine learning, implemented by a system of two neural networks competing against each other in a zero-sum game framework. They were first introduced by Ian Goodfellow *et al.* in 2014.

This technique can generate photographs that look authentic to human observers.

Method

One network is generative and one is discriminative. Typically, the generative network is taught to map from a latent space to a particular data distribution of interest, and the discriminative network is simultaneously taught to discriminate between instances from the true data distribution and synthesized instances produced by the generator. The generative network's training objective is to increase the error rate of the discriminative network (i.e., "fool" the discriminator network by producing novel synthesized instances that appear to have come from the true data distribution). These models are used for computer vision tasks.

In practice, a particular dataset serves as the training data for the discriminator. Training the discriminator involves presenting the discriminator with samples from the dataset and samples synthesized by the generator, and backpropagating from a binary classification loss. In order to produce a sample, typically the generator is seeded with a randomized input that is sampled from a predefined latent space (e.g., a multivariate normal distribution). Training the generator involves back-propagating the negation of the binary classification loss of the discriminator. The generator adjusts its parameters so that the training data and generated data cannot be distinguished by the discriminator model. The goal is to find a setting of parameters that makes generated data look like the training data to the discriminator network. In practice, the generator is typically a deconvolutional neural network, and the discriminator is a convolutional neural network.

The idea to infer models in a competitive setting (model versus discriminator) was first proposed by Li, Gauci and Gross in 2013. Their method is used for behavioral inference. It is termed Turing Learning, as the setting is akin to that of a Turing test.

Application

GANs can be used to produce samples of photorealistic images for the purposes of visualizing new interior/industrial design, shoes, bags and clothing items or items for computer games' scenes. These networks were reported to be used by Facebook. Recently, GANs have been able to model rudimentary patterns of motion in video. They have also been used to reconstruct 3D models of objects from images and to improve astronomical images.

Recurrent Neural Network

A recurrent neural network (RNN) is a class of artificial neural network where connections between units form a directed cycle. This creates an internal state of the network which allows it to exhibit dynamic temporal behavior. Unlike feedforward neural networks, RNNs can use their internal memory to process arbitrary sequences of inputs. This makes them applicable to tasks such as unsegmented connected handwriting recognition or speech recognition.

Architectures

Fully Recurrent Network

This is the basic architecture developed in the 1980s: a network of neuron-like units, each with a directed connection to every other unit. Each unit has a time-varying real-valued activation. Each connection has a modifiable real-valued weight. Some of the nodes are called input nodes, some output nodes, the rest hidden nodes. Most architectures below are special cases.

For supervised learning in discrete time settings, training sequences of real-valued input vectors become sequences of activations of the input nodes, one input vector at a time. At any given time step, each non-input unit computes its current activation as a nonlinear function of the weighted sum of the activations of all units from which it receives connections. There may be teacher-given target activations for some of the output units at certain time steps. For example, if the input sequence is a speech signal corresponding to a spoken digit, the final target output at the end of the sequence may be a label classifying the digit. For each sequence, its error is the sum of the deviations of all target signals from the corresponding activations computed by the network. For a training set of numerous sequences, the total error is the sum of the errors of all individual sequences. Algorithms for minimizing this error are mentioned in the section on training algorithms below.

In reinforcement learning settings, there is no teacher providing target signals for the RNN, instead a fitness function or reward function is occasionally used to evaluate the RNN's performance, which is influencing its input stream through output units connected to actuators affecting the environment. Again, compare the section on training algorithms below.

Recursive Neural Networks

A recursive neural network is created by applying the same set of weights recursively over a differentiable graph-like structure, by traversing the structure in topological order. Such networks are typically also trained by the reverse mode of automatic differentiation. They were introduced to learn distributed representations of structure, such as logical terms. A special case of recursive neural networks is the RNN itself whose structure corresponds to a linear chain. Recursive neural networks have been applied to natural language processing. The Recursive Neural Tensor Network uses a tensor-based composition function for all nodes in the tree.

Hopfield Network

The Hopfield network is of historic interest although it is not a general RNN, as it is not designed to process sequences of patterns. Instead it requires stationary inputs. It is a RNN in which all connections are symmetric. Invented by John Hopfield in 1982, it guarantees that its dynamics will converge. If the connections are trained using Hebbian learning then the Hopfield network can perform as robust content-addressable memory, resistant to connection alteration.

A variation on the Hopfield network is the bidirectional associative memory (BAM). The BAM has two layers, either of which can be driven as an input, to recall an association and produce an output on the other layer.

Elman Networks and Jordan Networks

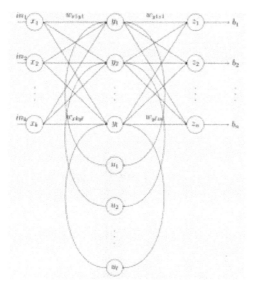

The Elman network

The following special case of the basic architecture above was employed by Jeff Elman. A three-layer network is used (arranged horizontally as x, y, and z in the illustration), with the addition of a set of "context units" (u in the illustration). There are connections from the middle (hidden) layer to these context units fixed with a weight of one. At each time step, the input is propagated in a standard feed-forward fashion, and then a learning rule is applied. The fixed back connections result in the context units always maintaining a copy of the previous values of the hidden units (since they propagate over the connections before the learning rule is applied). Thus the network can maintain a sort of state, allowing it to perform such tasks as sequence-prediction that are beyond the power of a standard multilayer perceptron.

Jordan networks, due to Michael I. Jordan, are similar to Elman networks. The context units are however fed from the output layer instead of the hidden layer. The context units in a Jordan network are also referred to as the state layer, and have a recurrent connection to themselves with no other nodes on this connection.

Elman and Jordan networks are also known as "simple recurrent networks" (SRN).

Elman network

$$h_t = \sigma_h(W_h x_t + U_h h_{t-1} + b_h)$$
$$y_t = \sigma_y(W_y h_t + b_y)$$

Jordan network

$$h_t = \sigma_h(W_h x_t + U_h y_{t-1} + b_h)$$
$$y_t = \sigma_y(W_y h_t + b_y)$$

Variables and functions

- x_t : input vector

- h_t : hidden layer vector

- y_t : output vector

- W, U and b : parameter matrices and vector

- σ_h and σ_y : Activation functions

Echo State Network

The echo state network (ESN) is a recurrent neural network with a sparsely connected random hidden layer. The weights of output neurons are the only part of the network that can change and be trained. ESN are good at reproducing certain time series. A variant for spiking neurons is known as liquid state machines.

Neural History Compressor

The vanishing gradient problem of automatic differentiation or backpropagation in neural networks was partially overcome in 1992 by an early generative model called the neural history compressor, implemented as an unsupervised stack of recurrent neural networks (RNNs). The RNN at the input level learns to predict its next input from the previous input history. Only unpredictable inputs of some RNN in the hierarchy become inputs to the next higher level RNN which therefore recomputes its internal state only rarely. Each higher level RNN thus learns a compressed representation of the information in the RNN below. This is done such that the input sequence can be precisely reconstructed from the sequence representation at the highest level. The system effectively minimises the description length or the negative logarithm of the probability of the data. If there is a lot of learnable predictability in the incoming data sequence, then the highest level RNN can use supervised learning to easily classify even deep sequences with very long time intervals between important events. In 1993, such a system already solved a "Very Deep Learning" task that requires more than 1000 subsequent layers in an RNN unfolded in time.

It is also possible to distill the entire RNN hierarchy into only two RNNs called the "conscious" chunker (higher level) and the "subconscious" automatizer (lower level). Once the chunker has learned to predict and compress inputs that are still unpredictable by the automatizer, then the automatizer can be forced in the next learning phase to predict or imitate through special additional units the hidden units of the more slowly changing chunker. This makes it easy for the automatizer to learn appropriate, rarely changing memories across very long time intervals. This in turn helps the automatizer to make many of its once unpredictable inputs predictable, such that the chunker can focus on the remaining still unpredictable events, to compress the data even further.

Long Short-term Memory

Numerous researchers now use a deep learning RNN called the long short-term memory (LSTM) network, published by Hochreiter & Schmidhuber in 1997. It is a deep learning system that unlike traditional RNNs doesn't have the vanishing gradient problem (compare the section on training algorithms below). LSTM is normally augmented by recurrent gates called forget gates. LSTM RNNs prevent backpropagated errors from vanishing or exploding. Instead errors can flow backwards through unlimited numbers of virtual layers in LSTM RNNs unfolded in space. That is, LSTM can learn "Very Deep Learning" tasks that require memories of events that happened thousands or even millions of discrete time steps ago. Problem-specific LSTM-like topologies can be evolved. LSTM works even when there are long delays, and it can handle signals that have a mix of low and high frequency components.

Today, many applications use stacks of LSTM RNNs and train them by Connectionist Temporal Classification (CTC) to find an RNN weight matrix that maximizes the probability of the label sequences in a training set, given the corresponding input sequences. CTC achieves both alignment and recognition. Around 2007, LSTM started to revolutionise speech recognition, outperforming traditional models in certain speech applications. In 2009, CTC-trained LSTM was the first RNN to win pattern recognition contests, when it won several competitions in connected handwriting recognition. In 2014, the Chinese search giant Baidu used CTC-trained RNNs to break the Switchboard Hub5'00 speech recognition benchmark, without using any traditional speech processing methods. LSTM also improved large-vocabulary speech recognition, text-to-speech synthesis, also for Google Android, and photo-real talking heads. In 2015, Google's speech recognition reportedly experienced a dramatic performance jump of 49% through CTC-trained LSTM, which is now available through Google voice search to all smartphone users.

LSTM has also become very popular in the field of natural language processing. Unlike previous models based on HMMs and similar concepts, LSTM can learn to recognise context-sensitive languages. LSTM improved machine translation, Language Modeling and Multilingual Language Processing. LSTM combined with convolutional neural networks (CNNs) also improved automatic image captioning and a plethora of other applications.

Gated Recurrent Unit

Gated recurrent unit is one of the recurrent neural network introduced in 2014.

Bi-directional RNN

Invented by Schuster & Paliwal in 1997, bi-directional RNN or BRNN use a finite sequence to predict or label each element of the sequence based on both the past and the future context of the element. This is done by concatenating the outputs of two RNN, one processing the sequence from left to right, the other one from right to left. The combined outputs are the predictions of the teacher-given target signals. This technique proved to be especially useful when combined with LSTM RNN.

Continuous-time RNN

A continuous time recurrent neural network (CTRNN) is a dynamical systems model of biological neural networks. A CTRNN uses a system of ordinary differential equations to model the effects on a neuron of the incoming spike train.

For a neuron i in the network with action potential y_i the rate of change of activation is given by:

$$\tau_i \dot{y}_i = -y_i + \sum_{j=1}^{n} w_{ji} \sigma(y_j - \Theta_j) + I_i(t)$$

Where:

- τ_i : Time constant of postsynaptic node

- y_i : Activation of postsynaptic node

- $\dot{y}_i$: Rate of change of activation of postsynaptic node

- w_{ji} : Weight of connection from pre to postsynaptic node

- $\sigma(x)$: Sigmoid of x e.g. $\sigma(x) = 1/(1+e^{-x})$.

- y_j : Activation of presynaptic node

- Θ_j : Bias of presynaptic node

- $I_i(t)$: Input (if any) to node

CTRNNs have frequently been applied in the field of evolutionary robotics, where they have been used to address, for example, vision, co-operation and minimally cognitive behaviour.

Note that by the Shannon sampling theorem, discrete time recurrent neural networks can be viewed as continuous time recurrent neural networks where the differential equation have transformed in an equivalent difference equation after that the postsynaptic node activation functions $y_i(t)$ have been low-pass filtered prior to sampling.

Hierarchical RNN

There are many instances of hierarchical RNN whose elements are connected in various ways to decompose hierarchical behavior into useful subprograms.

Recurrent Multilayer Perceptron

Generally, a Recurrent Multi-Layer Perceptron (RMLP) consists of a series of cascaded subnetworks, each of which consists of multiple layers of nodes. Each of these subnetworks is entirely feed-forward except for the last layer, which can have feedback connections among itself. Each of these subnets is connected only by feed forward connections.

Second Order RNN

Second order RNNs use higher order weights w_{ijk} instead of the standard w_{ij} weights, and inputs and states can be a product. This allows a direct mapping to a finite state machine both in training, stability, and representation. Long short-term memory is an example of this but has no such formal mappings or proof of stability.

Multiple Timescales Recurrent Neural Network (MTRNN) Model

MTRNN is a possible neural-based computational model that imitates to some extent the activity of the brain. It has the ability to simulate the functional hierarchy of the brain through self-organization that not only depends on spatial connection between neurons, but also on distinct types of neuron activities, each with distinct time properties. With such varied neuronal activities, continuous sequences of any set of behaviors are segmented into reusable primitives, which in turn are flexibly integrated into diverse sequential behaviors. The biological approval of such a type of hierarchy has been discussed on the memory-prediction theory of brain function by Jeff Hawkins in his book *On Intelligence*.

Pollack's Sequential Cascaded Networks

Neural Turing Machines

Neural Turing machine (NTMs) are a method of extending the capabilities of recurrent neural networks by coupling them to external memory resources, which they can interact with by attentional processes. The combined system is analogous to a Turing machine or Von Neumann architecture but is differentiable end-to-end, allowing it to be efficiently trained with gradient descent.

Neural Network Pushdown Automata

NNPDAs are similar to NTMs but tapes are replaced by analogue stacks that are differentiable and which are trained to control. In this way they are similar in complexity to recognizers of context free grammars (CFGs).

Bidirectional Associative Memory

First introduced by Kosko, BAM neural networks store associative data as a vector. The bi-directionality comes from passing information through a matrix and its transpose. Typically, bipolar encoding is preferred to binary encoding of the associative pairs. Recently, stochastic BAM models using Markov stepping were optimized for increased network stability and relevance to real-world applications.

Training

Gradient Descent

To minimize total error, gradient descent can be used to change each weight in proportion to the derivative of the error with respect to that weight, provided the non-linear activation functions are differentiable. Various methods for doing so were developed in the 1980s and early 1990s by Paul Werbos, Ronald J. Williams, Tony Robinson, Jürgen Schmidhuber, Sepp Hochreiter, Barak Pearlmutter, and others.

The standard method is called "backpropagation through time" or BPTT, and is a generalization of back-propagation for feed-forward networks, and like that method, is an instance of automatic differentiation in the reverse accumulation mode or Pontryagin's minimum principle. A more computationally expensive online variant is called "Real-Time Recurrent Learning" or RTRL, which is an instance of Automatic differentiation in the forward accumulation mode with stacked tangent vectors. Unlike BPTT this algorithm is *local in time but not local in space*.

In this context, *local in space* means that a unit's weight vector can be updated only using information stored in the connected units and the unit itself such that update complexity of a single unit is linear in the dimensionality of the weight vector. *Local in time* means that that the updates take place continually (on-line) and only depend on the most recent time step rather than on multiple time steps within a given time horizon as in BPTT. Biological neural networks appear to be local both with respect to time and space.

The downside of RTRL is that for recursively computing the partial derivatives, it has a time-complexity of O(number of hidden x number of weights) per time step for computing the Jacobian matrices, whereas BPTT only takes O(number of weights) per time step, at the cost, however, of storing all forward activations within the given time horizon.

There also is an online hybrid between BPTT and RTRL with intermediate complexity, and there are variants for continuous time. A major problem with gradient descent for standard RNN architectures is that error gradients vanish exponentially quickly with the size of the time lag between important events. The long short-term memory architecture together with a BPTT/RTRL hybrid learning method was introduced in an attempt to overcome these problems.

Moreover, the on-line algorithm called causal recursive BP (CRBP), implements and combines together BPTT and RTRL paradigms for locally recurrent network. It works with the most general locally recurrent networks. The CRBP algorithm can minimize the global error; this fact results in an improved stability of the algorithm, providing a unifying view on gradient calculation techniques for recurrent networks with local feedback.

An interesting approach to the computation of gradient information in RNNs with arbitrary architectures was proposed by Wan and Beaufays, is based on signal-flow graphs diagrammatic derivation to obtain the BPTT batch algorithm while, based on Lee theorem for networks sensitivity calculations, its fast online version was proposed by Campolucci, Uncini and Piazza.

Global Optimization Methods

Training the weights in a neural network can be modeled as a non-linear global optimization problem. A target function can be formed to evaluate the fitness or error of a particular weight vector as follows: First, the weights in the network are set according to the weight vector. Next, the network is evaluated against the training sequence. Typically, the sum-squared-difference between the predictions and the target values specified in the training sequence is used to represent the error of the current weight vector. Arbitrary global optimization techniques may then be used to minimize this target function.

The most common global optimization method for training RNNs is genetic algorithms, especially in unstructured networks.

Initially, the genetic algorithm is encoded with the neural network weights in a predefined manner where one gene in the chromosome represents one weight link, henceforth; the whole network is represented as a single chromosome. The fitness function is evaluated as follows: 1) each weight encoded in the chromosome is assigned to the respective weight link of the network; 2) the training set of examples is then presented to the network which propagates the input signals forward; 3) the mean-squared-error is returned to the fitness function; 4) this function will then drive the genetic selection process.

There are many chromosomes that make up the population; therefore, many different neural networks are evolved until a stopping criterion is satisfied. A common stopping scheme is: 1) when the neural network has learnt a certain percentage of the training data or 2) when the minimum value of the mean-squared-error is satisfied or 3) when the maximum number of training generations has been reached. The stopping criterion is evaluated by the fitness function as it gets the reciprocal of the mean-squared-error from each neural network during training. Therefore, the goal of the genetic algorithm is to maximize the fitness function, hence, reduce the mean-squared-error.

Other global (and/or evolutionary) optimization techniques may be used to seek a good set of weights such as simulated annealing or particle swarm optimization.

Related Fields and Models

RNNs may behave chaotically. In such cases, dynamical systems theory may be used for analysis.

Recurrent neural networks are in fact recursive neural networks with a particular structure: that of a linear chain. Whereas recursive neural networks operate on any hierarchical structure, combining child representations into parent representations, recurrent neural networks operate on the linear progression of time, combining the previous time step and a hidden representation into the representation for the current time step.

In particular, recurrent neural networks can appear as nonlinear versions of finite impulse response and infinite impulse response filters and also as a nonlinear autoregressive exogenous model (NARX).

Common RNN Libraries

- Apache Singa

- Caffe: Created by the Berkeley Vision and Learning Center (BVLC). It supports both CPU and GPU. Developed in C++, and has Python and MATLAB wrappers.

- Deeplearning4j: Deep learning in Java and Scala on multi-GPU-enabled Spark. A general-purpose deep learning library for the JVM production stack running on a C++ scientific computing engine. Allows the creation of custom layers. Integrates with Hadoop and Kafka.

- Keras

- Microsoft Cognitive Toolkit

- TensorFlow: Apache 2.0-licensed Theano-like library with support for CPU, GPU and Google's proprietary TPU, mobile

- Theano: The reference deep-learning library for Python with an API largely compatible with the popular NumPy library. Allows user to write symbolic mathematical expressions, then automatically generates their derivatives, saving the user from having to code gradients or backpropagation. These symbolic expressions are automatically compiled to CUDA code for a fast, on-the-GPU implementation.

- Torch: A scientific computing framework with wide support for machine learning algorithms, written in C and lua. The main author is Ronan Collobert.

Neural Network Software

Neural network software is used to simulate, research, develop, and apply artificial neural networks, software concepts adapted from biological neural networks, and, in some cases, a wider array of adaptive systems such as artificial intelligence and machine learning.

Simulators

Neural network simulators are software applications that are used to simulate the behavior of artificial or biological neural networks. They focus on one or a limited number of specific types of neural networks. They are typically stand-alone and not intended to produce general neural networks that can be integrated in other software. Simulators usually have some form of built-in visualization to monitor the training process. Some simulators also visualize the physical structure of the neural network.

Research Simulators

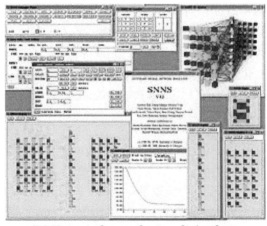

SNNS research neural network simulator

Historically, the most common type of neural network software was intended for researching neural network structures and algorithms. The primary purpose of this type of software is, through simulation, to gain a better understanding of the behavior and properties of neural networks. Today in the study of artificial neural networks, simulators have largely been replaced by more general component based development environments as research platforms.

Commonly used artificial neural network simulators include the Stuttgart Neural Network Simulator (SNNS), Emergent and Neural Lab.

In the study of biological neural networks however, simulation software is still the only available approach. In such simulators the physical biological and chemical properties of neural tissue, as well as the electromagnetic impulses between the neurons are studied.

Commonly used biological network simulators include Neuron, GENESIS, NEST and Brian.

Data Analysis Simulators

Unlike the research simulators, data analysis simulators are intended for practical applications of artificial neural networks. Their primary focus is on data mining and forecasting. Data analysis simulators usually have some form of preprocessing capabilities. Unlike the more general development environments data analysis simulators use a relatively simple static neural network that can be configured. A majority of the data analysis simulators on the market use backpropagating networks or self-organizing maps as their core. The advantage of this type of software is that it is relatively easy to use. Neural Designer is one example of a data analysis simulator.

Simulators for Teaching Neural Network Theory

When the Parallel Distributed Processing volumes were released in 1986-87, they provided some relatively simple software. The original PDP software did not require any programming skills, which led to its adoption by a wide variety of researchers in diverse fields. The original PDP software was developed into a more powerful package called PDP++, which in turn has become an even more powerful platform called Emergent. With each development, the software has become more powerful, but also more daunting for use by beginners.

In 1997, the tLearn software was released to accompany a book. This was a return to the idea of providing a small, user-friendly, simulator that was designed with the novice in mind. tLearn allowed basic feed forward networks, along with simple recurrent networks, both of which can be trained by the simple back propagation algorithm. tLearn has not been updated since 1999.

In 2011, the Basic Prop simulator was released. Basic Prop is a self-contained application, distributed as a platform neutral JAR file, that provides much of the same simple functionality as tLearn.

In 2012, Wintempla included a namespace called NN with a set of C++ classes to implement: feed forward networks, probabilistic neural networks and Kohonen networks. Neural Lab is based on Wintempla classes. Neural Lab tutorial and Wintempla tutorial explains some of these clases for neural networks. The main disadvantage of Wintempla is that it compiles only with Microsoft Visual Studio.

Development Environments

Development environments for neural networks differ from the software described above primarily on two accounts – they can be used to develop custom types of neural networks and they support deployment of the neural network outside the environment. In some cases they have advanced preprocessing, analysis and visualization capabilities.

Component Based

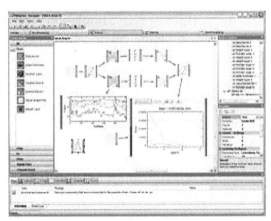

Peltarion Synapse component based development environment.

A more modern type of development environments that are currently favored in both industrial and scientific use are based on a component based paradigm. The neural network is constructed by connecting adaptive filter components in a pipe filter flow. This allows for greater flexibility as custom networks can be built as well as custom components used by the network. In many cases this allows a combination of adaptive and non-adaptive components to work together. The data flow is controlled by a control system which is exchangeable as well as the adaptation algorithms. The other important feature is deployment capabilities.

With the advent of component-based frameworks such as .NET and Java, component based development environments are capable of deploying the developed neural network to these frameworks as inheritable components. In addition some software can also deploy these components to several platforms, such as embedded systems.

Component based development environments include: Peltarion Synapse, NeuroDimension NeuroSolutions, Scientific Software Neuro Laboratory, and the LIONsolver integrated software. Free open source component based environments include Encog and Neuroph.

Criticism

A disadvantage of component-based development environments is that they are more complex than simulators. They require more learning to fully operate and are more complicated to develop.

Custom Neural Networks

The majority implementations of neural networks available are however custom implementations in various programming languages and on various platforms. Basic types of neural networks are simple to implement directly. There are also many programming libraries that contain neural network functionality and that can be used in custom implementations (such as tensorflow, theano, etc., typically providing bindings to languages such as python, C++, Java).

Standards

In order for neural network models to be shared by different applications, a common language is necessary. The Predictive Model Markup Language (PMML) has been proposed to address this need. PMML is an XML-based language which provides a way for applications to define and share neural network models (and other data mining models) between PMML compliant applications.

PMML provides applications a vendor-independent method of defining models so that proprietary issues and incompatibilities are no longer a barrier to the exchange of models between applications. It allows users to develop models within one vendor's application, and use other vendors' applications to visualize, analyze, evaluate or otherwise use the models. Previously, this was very difficult, but with PMML, the exchange of models between compliant applications is now straightforward.

PMMl Consumers and Producers

A range of products are being offered to produce and consume PMML. This ever-growing list includes the following neural network products:

- R: produces PMML for neural nets and other machine learning models via the package pmml.

- SAS Enterprise Miner: produces PMML for several mining models, including neural networks, linear and logistic regression, decision trees, and other data mining models.

- SPSS: produces PMML for neural networks as well as many other mining models.

- STATISTICA: produces PMML for neural networks, data mining models and traditional statistical models.

Machine Learning

Machine learning is the subfield of computer science that, according to Arthur Samuel in 1959, gives "computers the ability to learn without being explicitly programmed." Evolved from the study of pattern recognition and computational learning theory in artificial intelligence, machine learning explores the study and construction of algorithms that can learn from and make predictions on data – such algorithms overcome following strictly static program instructions by making data-driven predictions or decisions, through building a model from sample inputs. Machine learning is employed in a range of computing tasks where designing and programming explicit algorithms with good performance is difficult or unfeasible; example applications include email filtering, detection of network intruders or malicious insiders working towards a data breach, optical character recognition (OCR), learning to rank and computer vision.

Machine learning is closely related to (and often overlaps with) computational statistics, which also focuses on prediction-making through the use of computers. It has strong ties to mathematical optimization, which delivers methods, theory and application domains to the field. Machine learning is sometimes conflated with data mining, where the latter subfield focuses more on exploratory data analysis and is known as unsupervised learning. Machine learning can also be unsupervised and be used to learn and establish baseline behavioral profiles for various entities and then used to find meaningful anomalies.

Within the field of data analytics, machine learning is a method used to devise complex models and algorithms that lend themselves to prediction; in commercial use, this is known as predictive analytics. These analytical models allow researchers, data scientists, engineers, and analysts to "produce reliable, repeatable decisions and results" and uncover "hidden insights" through learning from historical relationships and trends in the data.

As of 2016, machine learning is a buzzword, and according to the Gartner hype cycle of 2016, at its peak of inflated expectations. Because finding patterns is hard, often not enough training data is available, and also because of the high expectations it often fails to deliver.

Overview

Tom M. Mitchell provided a widely quoted, more formal definition: "A computer program is said to learn from experience E with respect to some class of tasks T and performance measure P if its performance at tasks in T, as measured by P, improves with experience E." This definition is notable for its defining machine learning in fundamentally operational rather than cognitive terms, thus following Alan Turing's proposal in his paper "Computing Machinery and Intelligence", that the question "Can machines think?" be replaced with the question "Can machines do what we (as thinking entities) can do?". In the proposal he explores the various characteristics that could be possessed by a *thinking machine* and the various implications in constructing one.

Types of Problems and Tasks

Machine learning tasks are typically classified into three broad categories, depending on the nature of the learning "signal" or "feedback" available to a learning system. These are

- Supervised learning: The computer is presented with example inputs and their desired outputs, given by a "teacher", and the goal is to learn a general rule that maps inputs to outputs.

- Unsupervised learning: No labels are given to the learning algorithm, leaving it on its own to find structure in its input. Unsupervised learning can be a goal in itself (discovering hidden patterns in data) or a means towards an end (feature learning).

- Reinforcement learning: A computer program interacts with a dynamic environment in which it must perform a certain goal (such as driving a vehicle or playing a game against an opponent). The program is provided feedback in terms of rewards and punishments as it navigates its problem space.

Between supervised and unsupervised learning is semi-supervised learning, where the teacher gives an incomplete training signal: a training set with some (often many) of the target outputs missing. Transduction is a special case of this principle where the entire set of problem instances is known at learning time, except that part of the targets are missing.

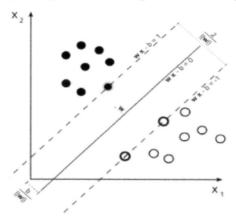

A support vector machine is a classifier that divides its input space into two regions, separated by a linear boundary. Here, it has learned to distinguish black and white circles

Among other categories of machine learning problems, learning to learn learns its own inductive bias based on previous experience. Developmental learning, elaborated for robot learning, generates its own sequences (also called curriculum) of learning situations to cumulatively acquire repertoires of novel skills through autonomous self-exploration and social interaction with human teachers and using guidance mechanisms such as active learning, maturation, motor synergies, and imitation.

Another categorization of machine learning tasks arises when one considers the desired *output* of a machine-learned system:

- In classification, inputs are divided into two or more classes, and the learner must produce a model that assigns unseen inputs to one or more (multi-label classification) of these classes. This is typically tackled in a supervised way. Spam filtering is an example of classification, where the inputs are email (or other) messages and the classes are "spam" and "not spam".

- In regression, also a supervised problem, the outputs are continuous rather than discrete.

- In clustering, a set of inputs is to be divided into groups. Unlike in classification, the groups are not known beforehand, making this typically an unsupervised task.

- Density estimation finds the distribution of inputs in some space.

- Dimensionality reduction simplifies inputs by mapping them into a lower-dimensional space. Topic modeling is a related problem, where a program is given a list of human language documents and is tasked to find out which documents cover similar topics.

History and Relationships to Other Fields

As a scientific endeavour, machine learning grew out of the quest for artificial intelligence. Already in the early days of AI as an academic discipline, some researchers were interested in having machines learn from data. They attempted to approach the problem with various symbolic methods, as well as what were then termed "neural networks"; these were mostly perceptrons and other models that were later found to be reinventions of the generalized linear models of statistics. Probabilistic reasoning was also employed, especially in automated medical diagnosis.

However, an increasing emphasis on the logical, knowledge-based approach caused a rift between AI and machine learning. Probabilistic systems were plagued by theoretical and practical problems of data acquisition and representation. By 1980, expert systems had come to dominate AI, and statistics was out of favor. Work on symbolic/knowledge-based learning did continue within AI, leading to inductive logic programming, but the more statistical line of research was now outside the field of AI proper, in pattern recognition and information retrieval. Neural networks research had been abandoned by AI and computer science around the same time. This line, too, was continued outside the AI/CS field, as "connectionism", by researchers from other disciplines including Hopfield, Rumelhart and Hinton. Their main success came in the mid-1980s with the reinvention of backpropagation.

Machine learning, reorganized as a separate field, started to flourish in the 1990s. The field changed its goal from achieving artificial intelligence to tackling solvable problems of a practical nature. It shifted focus away from the symbolic approaches it had inherited from AI, and toward methods and models borrowed from statistics and probability theory. It also benefited from the increasing availability of digitized information, and the possibility to distribute that via the Internet.

Machine learning and data mining often employ the same methods and overlap significantly, but while machine learning focuses on prediction, based on *known* properties learned from the training data, data mining focuses on the discovery of (previously) *unknown* properties in the data (this is the analysis step of Knowledge Discovery in Databases). Data mining uses many machine learning methods, but with different goals; on the other hand, machine learning also employs data mining methods as "unsupervised learning" or as a preprocessing step to improve learner accuracy. Much of the confusion between these two research communities (which do often have separate conferences and separate journals, ECML PKDD being a major exception) comes from the basic assumptions they work with: in machine learning, performance is usually evaluated with respect to the ability to *reproduce known* knowledge, while in Knowledge Discovery and Data Mining (KDD) the key task is the discovery of previously *unknown* knowledge. Evaluated with respect to known knowledge, an uninformed (unsupervised) method will easily be outperformed by other supervised methods, while in a typical KDD task, supervised methods cannot be used due to the unavailability of training data.

Machine learning also has intimate ties to optimization: many learning problems are formulated as minimization of some loss function on a training set of examples. Loss functions express the discrepancy between the predictions of the model being trained and the actual problem instances (for example, in classification, one wants to assign a label to instances, and models are trained to correctly predict the pre-assigned labels of a set examples). The difference between the two fields arises from the goal of generalization: while optimization algorithms can minimize the loss on a training set, machine learning is concerned with minimizing the loss on unseen samples.

Relation to Statistics

Machine learning and statistics are closely related fields. According to Michael I. Jordan, the ideas of machine learning, from methodological principles to theoretical tools, have had a long pre-history in statistics. He also suggested the term data science as a placeholder to call the overall field.

Leo Breiman distinguished two statistical modelling paradigms: data model and algorithmic model, wherein 'algorithmic model' means more or less the machine learning algorithms like Random forest.

Some statisticians have adopted methods from machine learning, leading to a combined field that they call *statistical learning*.

Theory

A core objective of a learner is to generalize from its experience. Generalization in this context is the ability of a learning machine to perform accurately on new, unseen examples/tasks after having experienced a learning data set. The training examples come from some generally unknown probability distribution (considered representative of the space of occurrences) and the learner has to build a general model about this space that enables it to produce sufficiently accurate predictions in new cases.

The computational analysis of machine learning algorithms and their performance is a branch of theoretical computer science known as computational learning theory. Because training sets are finite and the future is uncertain, learning theory usually does not yield guarantees of the performance of algorithms. Instead, probabilistic bounds on the performance are quite common. The bias–variance decomposition is one way to quantify generalization error.

For the best performance in the context of generalization, the complexity of the hypothesis should match the complexity of the function underlying the data. If the hypothesis is less complex than the function, then the model has underfit the data. If the complexity of the model is increased in response, then the training error decreases. But if the hypothesis is too complex, then the model is subject to overfitting and generalization will be poorer.

In addition to performance bounds, computational learning theorists study the time complexity and feasibility of learning. In computational learning theory, a computation is considered feasible if it can be done in polynomial time. There are two kinds of time complexity results. Positive results show that a certain class of functions can be learned in polynomial time. Negative results show that certain classes cannot be learned in polynomial time.

Approaches

Decision Tree Learning

Decision tree learning uses a decision tree as a predictive model, which maps observations about an item to conclusions about the item's target value.

Association Rule Learning

Association rule learning is a method for discovering interesting relations between variables in large databases.

Artificial Neural Networks

An artificial neural network (ANN) learning algorithm, usually called "neural network" (NN), is a learning algorithm that is inspired by the structure and functional aspects of biological neural networks. Computations are structured in terms of an interconnected group of artificial neurons, processing information using a connectionist approach to computation. Modern neural networks are non-linear statistical data modeling tools. They are usually used to model complex relationships between inputs and outputs, to find patterns in data, or to capture the statistical structure in an unknown joint probability distribution between observed variables.

Deep Learning

Falling hardware prices and the development of GPUs for personal use in the last few years have contributed to the development of the concept of Deep learning which consists of multiple hidden layers in an artificial neural network. This approach tries to model the way the human brain processes light and sound into vision and hearing. Some successful applications of deep learning are computer vision and speech recognition.

Inductive Logic Programming

Inductive logic programming (ILP) is an approach to rule learning using logic programming as a uniform representation for input examples, background knowledge, and hypotheses. Given an encoding of the known background knowledge and a set of examples represented as a logical database of facts, an ILP system will derive a hypothesized logic program that entails all positive and no negative examples. Inductive programming is a related field that considers any kind of programming languages for representing hypotheses (and not only logic programming), such as functional programs.

Support Vector Machines

Support vector machines (SVMs) are a set of related supervised learning methods used for classification and regression. Given a set of training examples, each marked as belonging to one of two categories, an SVM training algorithm builds a model that predicts whether a new example falls into one category or the other.

Clustering

Cluster analysis is the assignment of a set of observations into subsets (called *clusters*) so that observations within the same cluster are similar according to some predesignated criterion or criteria, while observations drawn from different clusters are dissimilar. Different clustering techniques make different assumptions on the structure of the data, often defined by some *similarity metric* and evaluated for example by *internal compactness* (similarity between members of the same cluster) and *separation* between different clusters. Other methods are based on *estimated density* and *graph connectivity*. Clustering is a method of unsupervised learning, and a common technique for statistical data analysis.

Bayesian Networks

A Bayesian network, belief network or directed acyclic graphical model is a probabilistic graphical model that represents a set of random variables and their conditional independencies via a directed acyclic graph (DAG). For example, a Bayesian network could represent the probabilistic relationships between diseases and symptoms. Given symptoms, the network can be used to compute the probabilities of the presence of various diseases. Efficient algorithms exist that perform inference and learning.

Reinforcement Learning

Reinforcement learning is concerned with how an *agent* ought to take *actions* in an *environment* so as to maximize some notion of long-term *reward*. Reinforcement learning algorithms attempt to find a *policy* that maps *states* of the world to the actions the agent ought to take in those states. Reinforcement learning differs from the supervised learning problem in that correct input/output pairs are never presented, nor sub-optimal actions explicitly corrected.

Representation Learning

Several learning algorithms, mostly unsupervised learning algorithms, aim at discovering better representations of the inputs provided during training. Classical examples include principal components analysis and cluster analysis. Representation learning algorithms often attempt to preserve the information in their input but transform it in a way that makes it useful, often as a pre-processing step before performing classification or predictions, allowing reconstruction of the inputs coming from the unknown data generating distribution, while not being necessarily faithful for configurations that are implausible under that distribution.

Manifold learning algorithms attempt to do so under the constraint that the learned representation is low-dimensional. Sparse coding algorithms attempt to do so under the constraint that the learned representation is sparse (has many zeros). Multilinear subspace learning algorithms aim to learn low-dimensional representations directly from tensor representations for multidimensional data, without reshaping them into (high-dimensional) vectors. Deep learning algorithms discover multiple levels of representation, or a hierarchy of features, with higher-level, more abstract features defined in terms of (or generating) lower-level features. It has been argued that an intelligent machine is one that learns a representation that disentangles the underlying factors of variation that explain the observed data.

Similarity and Metric Learning

In this problem, the learning machine is given pairs of examples that are considered similar and pairs of less similar objects. It then needs to learn a similarity function (or a distance metric function) that can predict if new objects are similar. It is sometimes used in Recommendation systems.

Sparse Dictionary Learning

In this method, a datum is represented as a linear combination of basis functions, and the coefficients are assumed to be sparse. Let x be a d-dimensional datum, D be a d by n matrix, where each column of D represents a basis function. r is the coefficient to represent x using D. Mathematically, sparse dictionary learning means solving $x \approx Dr$ where r is sparse. Generally speaking, n is assumed to be larger than d to allow the freedom for a sparse representation.

Learning a dictionary along with sparse representations is strongly NP-hard and also difficult to solve approximately. A popular heuristic method for sparse dictionary learning is K-SVD.

Sparse dictionary learning has been applied in several contexts. In classification, the problem is to determine which classes a previously unseen datum belongs to. Suppose a dictionary for each class has already been built. Then a new datum is associated with the class such that it's best sparsely represented by the corresponding dictionary. Sparse dictionary learning has also been applied in image de-noising. The key idea is that a clean image patch can be sparsely represented by an image dictionary, but the noise cannot.

Genetic Algorithms

A genetic algorithm (GA) is a search heuristic that mimics the process of natural selection, and uses methods such as mutation and crossover to generate new genotype in the hope of finding good solutions to a given problem. In machine learning, genetic algorithms found some uses in the 1980s and 1990s. Vice versa, machine learning techniques have been used to improve the performance of genetic and evolutionary algorithms.

Rule-based Machine Learning

Rule-based machine learning is a general term for any machine learning method that identifies, learns, or evolves `rules' to store, manipulate or apply, knowledge. The defining characteristic of a rule-based machine learner is the identification and utilization of a set of relational rules that collectively represent the knowledge captured by the system. This is in contrast to other machine learners that commonly identify a singular model that can be universally applied to any instance in order to make a prediction. Rule-based machine learning approaches include learning classifier systems, association rule learning, and artificial immune systems.

Learning Classifier Systems

Learning classifier systems (LCS) are a family of rule-based machine learning algorithms that combine a discovery component (e.g. typically a genetic algorithm) with a learning component (performing either supervised learning, reinforcement learning, or unsupervised learning). They seek to identify a set of context-dependent rules that collectively store and apply knowledge in a piecewise manner in order to make predictions.

Applications

Applications for machine learning include:

- Adaptive websites
- Affective computing
- Bioinformatics
- Brain-machine interfaces
- Cheminformatics

- Classifying DNA sequences
- Computational anatomy
- Computer vision, including object recognition
- Detecting credit card fraud
- Game playing
- Information retrieval
- Internet fraud detection
- Marketing
- Machine learning control
- Machine perception
- Medical diagnosis
- Economics
- Natural language processing
- Natural language understanding
- Optimization and metaheuristic
- Online advertising
- Recommender systems
- Robot locomotion
- Search engines
- Sentiment analysis (or opinion mining)
- Sequence mining
- Software engineering
- Speech and handwriting recognition
- Financial market analysis
- Structural health monitoring
- Syntactic pattern recognition
- User behavior analytics
- Translation

In 2006, the online movie company Netflix held the first "Netflix Prize" competition to find a program to better predict user preferences and improve the accuracy on its existing Cinematch movie recommendation algorithm by at least 10%. A joint team made up of researchers from AT&T

Labs-Research in collaboration with the teams Big Chaos and Pragmatic Theory built an ensemble model to win the Grand Prize in 2009 for $1 million. Shortly after the prize was awarded, Netflix realized that viewers' ratings were not the best indicators of their viewing patterns ("everything is a recommendation") and they changed their recommendation engine accordingly.

In 2010 The Wall Street Journal wrote about money management firm Rebellion Research's use of machine learning to predict economic movements. The article describes Rebellion Research's prediction of the financial crisis and economic recovery.

In 2012 co-founder of Sun Microsystems Vinod Khosla predicted that 80% of medical doctors jobs would be lost in the next two decades to automated machine learning medical diagnostic software.

In 2014 it has been reported that a machine learning algorithm has been applied in Art History to study fine art paintings, and that it may have revealed previously unrecognized influences between artists.

Model Assessments

Classification machine learning models can be validated by accuracy estimation techniques like the Holdout method, which splits the data in a training and test set (conventionally 2/3 training set and 1/3 test set designation) and evaluates the performance of the training model on the test set. In comparison, the N-fold-cross-validation method randomly splits the data in k subsets where the k-1 instances of the data are used to train the model while the kth instance is used to test the predictive ability of the training model. In addition to the holdout and cross-validation methods, bootstrap, which samples n instances with replacement from the dataset, can be used to assess model accuracy. In addition to accuracy, sensitivity and specificity (True Positive Rate: TPR and True Negative Rate: TNR, respectively) can provide modes of model assessment. Similarly False Positive Rate (FPR) as well as the False Negative Rate (FNR) can be computed. Receiver operating characteristic (ROC) along with the accompanying Area Under the ROC Curve (AUC) offer additional tools for classification model assessment. Higher AUC is associated with a better performing model.

Ethics

Machine Learning poses a host of ethical questions. Systems which are trained on datasets collected with biases may exhibit these biases upon use, thus digitizing cultural prejudices. Responsible collection of data thus is a critical part of machine learning.

Because language contains biases, machines trained on language corpora will necessarily also learn bias.

Perceptron

In machine learning, the perceptron is an algorithm for supervised learning of binary classifiers (functions that can decide whether an input, represented by a vector of numbers, belongs to some specific class or not). It is a type of linear classifier, i.e. a classification algorithm that makes its predictions based on a linear predictor function combining a set of weights with the feature vector. The algorithm allows for online learning, in that it processes elements in the training set one at a time.

The perceptron algorithm dates back to the late 1950s; its first implementation, in custom hardware, was one of the first artificial neural networks to be produced.

History

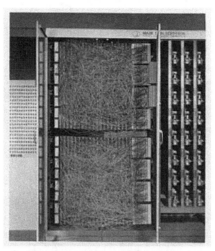

The Mark I Perceptron machine was the first implementation of the perceptron algorithm. The machine was connected to a camera that used 20×20 cadmium sulfide photocells to produce a 400-pixel image. The main visible feature is a patchboard that allowed experimentation with different combinations of input features. To the right of that are arrays of potentiometers that implemented the adaptive weights

The perceptron algorithm was invented in 1957 at the Cornell Aeronautical Laboratory by Frank Rosenblatt, funded by the United States Office of Naval Research. The perceptron was intended to be a machine, rather than a program, and while its first implementation was in software for the IBM 704, it was subsequently implemented in custom-built hardware as the "Mark 1 perceptron". This machine was designed for image recognition: it had an array of 400 photocells, randomly connected to the "neurons". Weights were encoded in potentiometers, and weight updates during learning were performed by electric motors.

In a 1958 press conference organized by the US Navy, Rosenblatt made statements about the perceptron that caused a heated controversy among the fledgling AI community; based on Rosenblatt's statements, *The New York Times* reported the perceptron to be "the embryo of an electronic computer that [the Navy] expects will be able to walk, talk, see, write, reproduce itself and be conscious of its existence."

Although the perceptron initially seemed promising, it was quickly proved that perceptrons could not be trained to recognise many classes of patterns. This caused the field of neural network research to stagnate for many years, before it was recognised that a feedforward neural network with two or more layers (also called a multilayer perceptron) had far greater processing power than perceptrons with one layer (also called a single layer perceptron). Single layer perceptrons are only capable of learning linearly separable patterns; in 1969 a famous book entitled *Perceptrons* by Marvin Minsky and Seymour Papert showed that it was impossible for these classes of network to learn an XOR function. It is often believed that they also conjectured (incorrectly) that a similar result would hold for a multi-layer perceptron network. However, this is not true, as both Minsky and Papert already knew that multi-layer perceptrons were capable of producing an XOR function. Three years later Stephen Grossberg published a series of papers introducing networks capable of modelling differential, contrast-enhancing and XOR functions. (The papers were published in 1972 and 1973, see e.g.:*Grossberg (1973). "Contour enhancement, short-term memory, and constancies in reverberating neural networks" (PDF). Studies in Applied Mathematics. 52: 213–257.*). Nevertheless, the often-miscited Minsky/Papert text caused a significant decline in interest and funding of neural network research. It took ten more years until neural network research experienced a resurgence in the 1980s. This text was reprinted in 1987 as "Perceptrons - Expanded Edition" where some errors in the original text are shown and corrected.

The kernel perceptron algorithm was already introduced in 1964 by Aizerman et al. Margin bounds guarantees were given for the Perceptron algorithm in the general non-separable case first by Freund and Schapire (1998), and more recently by Mohri and Rostamizadeh (2013) who extend previous results and give new L1 bounds.

Definition

In the modern sense, the perceptron is an algorithm for learning a binary classifier: a function that maps its input x (a real-valued vector) to an output value $f(x)$ (a single binary value):

$$f(x) = \begin{cases} 1 & \text{if } w \cdot x + b > 0 \\ 0 & \text{otherwise} \end{cases}$$

where w is a vector of real-valued weights, $w \cdot x$ is the dot product $\sum_{i=1}^{m} w_i x_i$, where m is the number of inputs to the perceptron and b is the *bias*. The bias shifts the decision boundary away from the origin and does not depend on any input value.

The value of $f(x)$ (0 or 1) is used to classify x as either a positive or a negative instance, in the case of a binary classification problem. If b is negative, then the weighted combination of inputs must produce a positive value greater than $|b|$ in order to push the classifier neuron over the 0 threshold. Spatially, the bias alters the position (though not the orientation) of the decision boundary. The perceptron learning algorithm does not terminate if the learning set is not linearly separable. If the vectors are not linearly separable learning will never reach a point where all vectors are classified properly. The most famous example of the perceptron's inability to solve problems with linearly nonseparable vectors is the Boolean exclusive-or problem. The solution spaces of decision boundaries for all binary functions and learning behaviors are studied in the reference.

In the context of neural networks, a perceptron is an artificial neuron using the Heaviside step function as the activation function. The perceptron algorithm is also termed the single-layer perceptron, to distinguish it from a multilayer perceptron, which is a misnomer for a more complicated neural network. As a linear classifier, the single-layer perceptron is the simplest feedforward neural network.

Learning Algorithm

Below is an example of a learning algorithm for a (single-layer) perceptron. For multilayer perceptrons, where a hidden layer exists, more sophisticated algorithms such as backpropagation must be used. Alternatively, methods such as the delta rule can be used if the function is non-linear and differentiable, although the one below will work as well.

When multiple perceptrons are combined in an artificial neural network, each output neuron operates independently of all the others; thus, learning each output can be considered in isolation.

Definitions

We first define some variables:

- $y = f(\mathbf{z})$ denotes the *output* from the perceptron for an input vector $\mathbf{z}$.

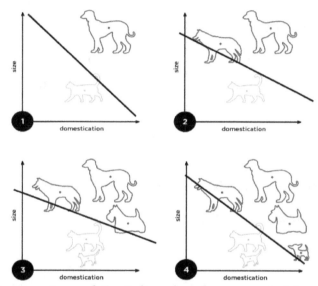

A diagram showing a perceptron updating its linear boundary as more training examples are added.

- $D = \{(\mathbf{x}_1, d_1), \ldots, (\mathbf{x}_s, d_s)\}$ is the *training set* of s samples, where:

  o $\mathbf{x}_j$ is the n-dimensional input vector.

  o d_j is the desired output value of the perceptron for that input.

We show the values of the features as follows:

- $x_{j,i}$ is the value of the ith feature of the jth training *input vector*.

- $x_{j,0} = 1$.

To represent the weights:

- w_i is the ith value in the *weight vector*, to be multiplied by the value of the ith input feature.

- Because $x_{j,0} = 1$, the w_0 is effectively a bias that we use instead of the bias constant b.

To show the time-dependence of w, we use:

- $w_i(t)$ is the weight i at time t.

Unlike other linear classification algorithms such as logistic regression, there is no need for a *learning rate* in the perceptron algorithm. This is because multiplying the update by any constant simply rescales the weights but never changes the sign of the prediction.

Steps

1. Initialize the weights and the threshold. Weights may be initialized to 0 or to a small random value. In the example below, we use 0.

2. For each example j in our training set D, perform the following steps over the input $\mathbf{x}_j$ and desired output d_j :

    a. Calculate the actual output:

    $$y_j(t) = f[\mathbf{w}(t)\cdot\mathbf{x}_j]$$
    $$= f[w_0(t)x_{j,0} + w_1(t)x_{j,1} + w_2(t)x_{j,2} + \cdots + w_n(t)x_{j,n}]$$

    b. Update the weights:

    $w_i(t+1) = w_i(t) + (d_j - y_j(t))x_{j,i}$, for all features $0 \le i \le n$.

3. For offline learning, the step 2 may be repeated until the iteration error $\dfrac{1}{s}\sum_{j=1}^{s}|d_j - y_j(t)|$ is less than a user-specified error threshold γ, or a predetermined number of iterations have been completed.

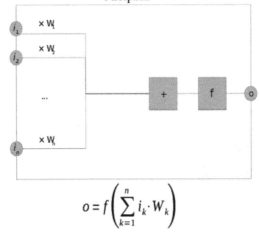

Perceptron

$$o = f\left(\sum_{k=1}^{n} i_k \cdot W_k\right)$$

The appropriate weights are applied to the inputs, and the resulting weighted sum passed to a function that produces the output o

The algorithm updates the weights after steps 2a and 2b. These weights are immediately applied to a pair in the training set, and subsequently updated, rather than waiting until all pairs in the training set have undergone these steps.

Convergence

The perceptron is a linear classifier, therefore it will never get to the state with all the input vectors classified correctly if the training set D is not linearly separable, i.e. if the positive examples can not be separated from the negative examples by a hyperplane. In this case, no "approximate" solution will be gradually approached under the standard learning algorithm, but instead learning will fail completely. Hence, if linear separability of the training set is not known a priori, one of the training variants below should be used.

But if the training set *is* linearly separable, then the perceptron is guaranteed to converge, and there is an upper bound on the number of times the perceptron will adjust its weights during the training.

Suppose that the input vectors from the two classes can be separated by a hyperplane with a margin γ, i.e. there exists a weight vector $\mathbf{w}, \| \mathbf{w} \| = 1$, and a bias term b such that $\mathbf{w} \cdot \mathbf{x}_j > \gamma$ for all $j : d_j = 1$ and $\mathbf{w} \cdot \mathbf{x}_j < -\gamma$ for all $j : d_j = 0$. And also let R denote the maximum norm of an input vector. Novikoff (1962) proved that in this case the perceptron algorithm converges after making $O(R^2 / \gamma^2)$ updates. The idea of the proof is that the weight vector is always adjusted by a bounded amount in a direction with which it has a negative dot product, and thus can be bounded above by $O\left(\sqrt{t}\right)$ where t is the number of changes to the weight vector. But it can also be bounded below by $O(t)$ because if there exists an (unknown) satisfactory weight vector, then every change makes progress in this (unknown) direction by a positive amount that depends only on the input vector.

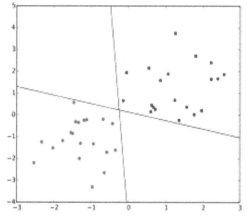

Two classes of points, and two of the infinitely many linear boundaries that separate them. Even though the boundaries are at nearly right angles to one another, the perceptron algorithm has no way of choosing between them.

While the perceptron algorithm is guaranteed to converge on *some* solution in the case of a linearly separable training set, it may still pick *any* solution and problems may admit many solutions of varying quality. The *perceptron of optimal stability*, nowadays better known as the linear support vector machine, was designed to solve this problem.

Variants

The pocket algorithm with ratchet (Gallant, 1990) solves the stability problem of perceptron learning by keeping the best solution seen so far "in its pocket". The pocket algorithm then returns the solution in the pocket, rather than the last solution. It can be used also for non-separable data sets, where the aim is to find a perceptron with a small number of misclassifications. However, these solutions appear purely stochastically and hence the pocket algorithm neither approaches them gradually in the course of learning, nor are they guaranteed to show up within a given number of learning steps.

The Maxover algorithm (Wendemuth, 1995) is "robust" in the sense that it will converge regardless of (prior) knowledge of linear separability of the data set. In the linear separable case, it will solve the training problem – if desired, even with optimal stability (maximum margin between the classes). For non-separable data sets, it will return a solution with a small number of misclassifications. In all cases, the algorithm gradually approaches the solution in the course of learning, without memorizing previous states and without stochastic jumps. Convergence is to global optimality for separable data sets and to local optimality for non-separable data sets.

In separable problems, perceptron training can also aim at finding the largest separating margin between the classes. The so-called perceptron of optimal stability can be determined by means of iterative training and optimization schemes, such as the Min-Over algorithm (Krauth and Mezard, 1987) or the AdaTron (Anlauf and Biehl, 1989)) . AdaTron uses the fact that the corresponding quadratic optimization problem is convex. The perceptron of optimal stability, together with the kernel trick, are the conceptual foundations of the support vector machine.

The α -perceptron further used a pre-processing layer of fixed random weights, with thresholded output units. This enabled the perceptron to classify analogue patterns, by projecting them into a binary space. In fact, for a projection space of sufficiently high dimension, patterns can become linearly separable.

Another way to solve nonlinear problems without using multiple layers is to use higher order networks (sigma-pi unit). In this type of network, each element in the input vector is extended with each pairwise combination of multiplied inputs (second order). This can be extended to an n-order network.

It should be kept in mind, however, that the best classifier is not necessarily that which classifies all the training data perfectly. Indeed, if we had the prior constraint that the data come from equi-variant Gaussian distributions, the linear separation in the input space is optimal, and the nonlinear solution is overfitted.

Other linear classification algorithms include Winnow, support vector machine and logistic regression.

Multiclass Perceptron

Like most other techniques for training linear classifiers, the perceptron generalizes naturally to multiclass classification. Here, the input x and the output y are drawn from arbitrary sets. A feature representation function $f(x, y)$ maps each possible input/output pair to a finite-dimensional real-valued feature vector. As before, the feature vector is multiplied by a weight vector w, but now the resulting score is used to choose among many possible outputs:

$$\hat{y} = \operatorname{argmax}_y f(x, y) \cdot w.$$

$\approx$ Learning again iterates over the examples, predicting an output for each, leaving the weights unchanged when the predicted output matches the target, and changing them when it does not. The update becomes:

$$w_{t+1} = w_t + f(x, y) - f(x, \hat{y}).$$

This multiclass feedback formulation reduces to the original perceptron when x is a real-valued vector, y is chosen from $\{0,1\}$, and $f(x,y) = yx.$.

For certain problems, input/output representations and features can be chosen so that $\text{argmax}_y f(x,y) \cdot w$ can be found efficiently even though y is chosen from a very large or even infinite set.

In recent years, perceptron training has become popular in the field of natural language processing for such tasks as part-of-speech tagging and syntactic parsing (Collins, 2002).

In a progressive simplification of single neuron models, we arrived at the McCulloch-Pitts neuron model which takes inputs from many neurons and produces a single output. If the net effect of the external inputs is greater than a threshold, the neuron goes into excited state (1), else it remains in its resting state (0).

Using this model, in 1943, its inventors Warren S. McCulloch, a neuroscientist, and Walter Pitts, a logician, set out to construct a model of brain function. Note that it was the time of World War- II. It was also a time when use of computing power was being tested for the first time on a large scale for war purposes – for calculating missile trajectories and breaking enemy codes. T he power of com-puting technology was just being realized by the world. Therefore it was natural to think of brain as a computer. Since the digital computer works on the basis of Boolean algebra, McCulloch and Pitts thought if it is possible for the brain also to use some form of Boolean algebra.

Since the MP neurons are binary units it seemed worthwhile to check if the basic logical operations can be performed by these neurons. McCulloch and Pitts quickly showed that the MP neuron can implement the basic logic gates AND, OR and NOT simply by proper choice of the weights:

OR Gate

The truth table of an OR gate is:

X1	X2	Y
0	0	0
0	1	1
1	0	1
1	1	1

Note that the function below, which represents a MP neuron with two inputs, x_1 and x_2, implements an OR gate.

$$y = g(x_1 + x_2 - b)$$

where b = 0.5; g(.) is the step function; $x_1, x_2 \in \{\ ,1\}$. Actually any value of the bias term b, $0 < b < 1$, should work.

AND Gate

The truth table of an AND gate is:

X1	X2	Y
0	0	0
0	1	0
1	0	0
1	1	1

Note that the function below implements an AND gate.

$$y = g(x_1 + x_2 - b)$$

Where $b = 1.5; g(.)$ is the step function; $x_1, x_2 \in \{0,1\}$. Actually any value of the bias term b, $1 < b < 2$, should work.

NOT Gate

$$y = g(-x + 0.5)$$

The truth table of a NOT gate is:

X	Y
0	1
1	0

Note that the function below implements a NOT gate.

$$y = g(-x + 0.5)$$

More generally, in $y = g(-x + b)$ any value of b in, $0 < b < 1$, would give a NOT gate.

Thus it became clear that by connecting properly designed MP neurons in specific architectures, any complex Boolean circuit can be constructed. Thus we have a theory of how brain can perform logical operations. McCulloch and Pitts explained their ideas in a paper titled, "A logical calculus of the ideas immanent in nervous activity" which appeared in the Bulletin of Mathematical Biophysics.

Although the idea of considering neurons as logic gates and the brain itself as a large Boolean circuit is quite tempting, it does not satisfy other important requirements of a good theory of the brain. There are some crucial differences between the brain and a digital computer (Table).

Table: Difference between the brain and a digital Computer

Property	Computer	Brain
Shape	2d Sheets of inorganic matter	3d volume of organic matter
Power	Powered by DC mains	Powered by ATP
Signal	Digital	pulsed
Clock	Centralized clock	No centralized clock
Clock speed	Gigahertz	100s of Hz

Fault tolerance	Highly fault-sensitive	Very fault-tolerant
Performance	By programming	By learning

Thus there are some fundamental differences between the computer and the brain. The signals used in the two systems are very different. There is no centralized clock in the brain. Each neuron fires at its own frequency which further changes with time. A brain is very fault tolerant which can be seen by the manner in which a stroke patient recovers. Most importantly a computer has to be programmed whereas the brain can learn by a progressive trial-and-error process.

These considerations led to the feeling that something is wrong with the McCulloch-Pitts approach to the brain.

As an answer to the above need, Frank Rosenblatt developed the Perceptron in 1957. A Perceptron is essentially a network of MP neurons.

Thus a Perceptron maps an m-dimensional input vector, onto a n-dimensional output vector. A distinct feature of a Perceptron is that the weights are not pre-calculated as in a MP neuron but are adjusted by a iterative process called training. The general approach to training, not only of a Perceptron, but of a larger class of neural networks (feedforward networks which will be defined later) is depicted in the figure below.

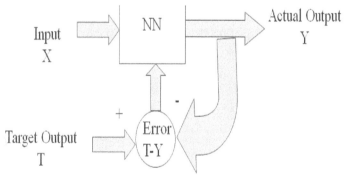

Training a neural network

The network is initialized with random weights

When an input X is presented to a neural network (NN), it responds with an output vector Y. Since the weights are random, the network output is likely to be wrong and therefore different from a Desired or a Target output T. Error defined as E = T-Y, is used to adjust the weights in the Perceptron (or NN in general) in such a way that the next time when X is presented to the network, the response Y is likely to be closer to T than before. This iterative procedure is continued with a large number of patterns until the error is minimum on all patterns.

The mechanism by which the weights are adjusted as a function of the error is called the learning rule.

The learning rule can vary depending on the precise architectural details of the Neural Network (NN) used in the above scheme.

Instead of directly taking up the task of deriving the learning rule for a Perceptron, let us begin with a very simple neuron model and derive the learning rule. In the process, we would introduce a few terms. The same procedure, with all its jargon, will be used to derive the learning rule for more complex architectures.

Case 1: Linear Neuron model: $\mathbf{y} = w^{\mathbf{T}}x$

Procedure to find the weights:

1) Noniterative , 2) Iterative

Output Error:

$$E = \frac{1}{2}\sum_{n}\left(y(p) - w^{T}x(p)\right)^{2}$$

$$\nabla_{w}E = \sum_{p}\left(-x(p)\right)\left(y(p) - w^{T}x(p)\right) = 0$$

1) Noniterative:

Pseudoinverse:

Let

$$X = \begin{bmatrix} x(1) \\ \cdot \\ \cdot \\ x(N) \end{bmatrix} = \begin{bmatrix} x_{1}(1) & x_{m}(1) \\ & \\ x_{1}(N) & x_{m}(N) \end{bmatrix}_{NXm}$$

$$Y = XW$$

$$w = [w_{1} \ \dots \ w_{m}]^{T}$$

$$y = [y(1) \ \dots \ y(N)]^{T}$$

$$d = [d(1) \ \dots \ d(N)]^{T}$$

$$E = (1/2)(d - XW)^{T}(d - XW) = (1/2)d^{T}d - (x^{T}d)^{T}w + (1/2)w^{T}(X^{T}X)w$$

$$W = (X^{T}X)^{-1}X^{T}d$$

$$R_{x} = (X^{T}X) \qquad correlation\ matrix$$

$$r_{xd} = X^{T}d \qquad cross-correlationmatrix$$

$$(X^{T}X)^{-1} \qquad pseudo-inverse$$

1) Iterative:

   a) Steepest Descent

$$w(t+1) = w(t) + \eta\sum_{p}(x(p))(d(p) - w^{T}x(p))$$

$$w(t+1) = w(t) + \eta\left(r_{xd} - R_{x}\ w(t)\right)$$

In the method of steepest descent, all the training data is used at the same time (packed into R_{x} and r_{xd}) to update every single weight. This can involve a large memory requirement and can be computationally expensive.

a) Least Mean Square Rule

$$w(t+1) = w(t) + (x(p))(d(p) - w^T x(p))$$

Also called the Delta Rule, Widrow-Hoff Rule.

Note that the key difference between the steepest descent rule above and the delta rule is the absence of summation over all training patterns in the latter.

In this case the weight vector does not smoothly converge on the final solution. Instead, it performs a random walk around the final solution and converges only in a least square sense.

Issues:

1. Convergence

1a. Shape of Error function, E (Single minimum for quadratic Error function)

Note that the dominant term in the error function of eqn. is a quadratic form associated with the correlation matrix, R_x.

Since R_x is a positive definite matrix the error function always has a unique minimum. It also has real, positive eigenvalues (λ_i).

1b. Effect of eigenvalues of correlation matrix

Condition number: $\lambda_{max} / \lambda_{min}$

where λ_{max} is the largest eigenvalue and λ_{min} is the smallest eigenvalue of the correlation matrix R_x.

Slows down the descent over the error function if the condition number is too large

1. The need to choose η.

    Large $\eta \rightarrow$ oscillations, instability

    Small $\eta \rightarrow$ slow convergence

    Bounds over the learning rate, η:

$$0 < \eta < 2/(\eta_{max})$$

Proof:

$$R_x = (X^T X) \qquad \text{correlation matrix}$$
$$r_{xd} = X^T d \qquad \text{cross-correlation matrix}$$
$$(X^T X)^{-1} \qquad \text{pseudo-inverse}$$
$$E = (1/2)(d - XW)^T (d - XW) = (1/2)d^T d - (X^T d)^T w + (1/2)w^T (X^T X)w$$
$$= (1/2)d^T d - r^T_{xd} w + (1/2)w^T (R_x)w$$

Final value of w, $w* = R_x^{-1} r_{xd}$

$$E = Emin + (1/2)(w-w*)^T R_x (w-w*)$$
$$\text{Grad}(E) = R_x(w-w*)$$
$$\text{Delta } w = -\eta \text{ grad}(E)$$
$$= -\eta \; w(t+1) = w(t) - \eta R_x(w(t)-w*)$$
$$w(t+1)-w* = (I-\eta R_x)(w(t)-w*)$$

$$\text{Let, } v(t) = (w(t)-w*)$$
$$v(t+1) = (I - \eta R_x) v(t)$$

Let $v' = Qv$, where Q is an orthogonal matrix that diagonalizes R_x

$$v'(t+1) = (I-\eta D)v'(t)$$

$$D = \begin{bmatrix} \lambda_1 & 0 & 0 & 0 \\ 0 & \lambda_2 & 0 & 0 \\ 0 & 0 & \ddots & 0 \\ 0 & 0 & 0 & \lambda_n \end{bmatrix}$$

If we consider the individual components, v_i, of eqn. above,

$$v_i(t+1) = (1-\eta\lambda_i)v_i(t)$$

The condition for stability of the last equation, is
$|1-\eta\lambda_i| < 1$. Let us consider the two possible cases of this inequality

a) $1-\eta\lambda_i < 1 \rightarrow \eta > 0$ which is trivial.

b) $-(1-\eta\lambda_i) < 1 \rightarrow \eta < 2/\lambda_i$ for all i.

Therefore,

$$\eta < 2/\lambda_{max}$$

3. The need to reduce η with time:

There are obvious tradeoffs between use of a large vs. small η. Large η speeds up learning but can be unstable. Small η is stable but results in slower learning.

Therefore, it is desirable to begin with a large η and reduce it with time.

Learning rate variation schedules:
$$\text{a)} \eta = c/n; \quad \text{b)} \eta = \eta_o/(1+(n/\tau))$$

Case 2: Perceptron: MP Neuron which has Sigmoid Nonlinearity

With the hard-limiting or threshold nonlinearity the neuron acts as a classifier.

Final solution is not unique.

Convergence only if linearly separable.

$$y = g(\sum_{i=1}^{n} w_i x_i - b)$$

Hardlimiter characteristics:

$$g(v) = 1, v \geq 0$$
$$= 0, v < 0$$

For a Perceptron with a single output neuron, the regions corresponding to the 2 classes are separated by a hyperplane given by:

$$\sum w_i x_i - b = 0$$

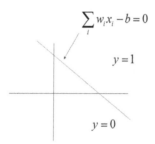

Classification by a perceptron

In other words, a Perceptron classifies input patterns by dividing the input space into two semi-infinite regions using a hyperplane.

Perceptron Learning Rule

It is also called the LMS Rule or Delta Rule or Widrow-Hoff Rule

The steps involved in Perceptron learning are as follows:

1. Initialization of weights: Set the initial values of the weights to 0. w(0) = 0.

2. Present the p'th training pattern, x, and calculate the network output, y.

3. Using the desired output, d, for the input pattern x, adjust the weights by a small amount using the following learning rule:

$$w(t+1) = w(t) + \eta[d(t) - y(t)]x(t)$$
where,
$$d(n) = +1, x(t) \in C1$$
$$d(n) = -1, x(t) \in C2$$

4. Go back to step 2 and continue until the network output error, e = d-y, is 0 for all patterns.

The above training process will converge after N_{max} iterations where,

$$\alpha = \min_{x(n) \in C1} w_0^T x(n)$$

$$\beta = \max_{x(k) \in C1} \| x(k) \|^2$$

$$N^{max} = \beta \| w_0 \|^2 / \alpha$$

Range of η:

$0 < \eta < 1$

- Averaging of past inputs leads to stable weight dynamics, which requires small η

- Fast adaptation requires large η

Learning rule can also be derived from an error function:

$$E = \frac{1}{2} \sum_p [(d_p - y_p)^2]$$

where E denotes the squared error over all patterns.

The learning rule may be derived by performing gradient descent over the error function.

Gradient of Error:

$$\Delta w = -\eta \nabla_w E$$

$$\Delta w_i = -\eta \frac{\partial E}{\partial w_i}$$

$$\frac{\partial E}{\partial w_i} = -[d-y]\frac{\partial y}{\partial w_i} = -[d-y]g'x_i$$

The last term in the above equation has g', which is zero everywhere except at the origin if g is a hardlimiting nonlinearity. But if we take a smoother version of g(), which saturate at +1 and -1, like the tanh() function, the learning rule becomes,

$$\Delta w_i = \eta [d-y]g'x_i$$

Since g' > 0 always for tanh() function, we can absorb it into h, considering it as a quantity that varies with x. We then have,

$$\Delta w_i = \eta'[d-y]x_i$$

Which is identical to the Perceptron learning rule given in eqn. above.

Features of Perceptron:

1) The Perceptrons can only classify linearly separable classes.

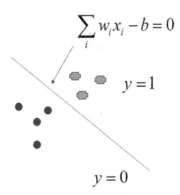

Classification of linear separable classes by a perceptron

2) When the training data is linearly separable, there can be an infinite number of solutions.

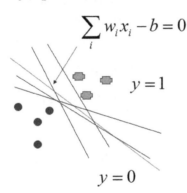

Solutions to classify linear separable classes by a perceptron

Critique of Perceptrons:

- Perceptrons cannot even solve simple problems like Xor problem

- Linear model: Can only discriminate linearly separable classes

- Even the multi-layered versions may be afflicted by these weaknesses (Minsky & Papert, 1969)

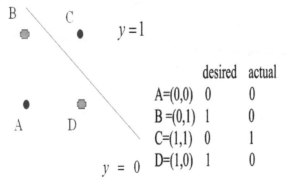

Inability to solve Xor by a perceptron

Multilayer Perceptron

A multilayer perceptron (MLP) is a feedforward artificial neural network model that maps sets of input data onto a set of appropriate outputs. An MLP consists of multiple layers of nodes in a directed graph, with each layer fully connected to the next one. Except for the input nodes, each node is a neuron (or processing element) with a nonlinear activation function. MLP utilizes a supervised learning technique called backpropagation for training the network. MLP is a modification of the standard linear perceptron and can distinguish data that is not linearly separable.

Theory

Activation Function

If a multilayer perceptron has a linear activation function in all neurons, that is, a linear function that maps the weighted inputs to the output of each neuron, then it is easily proven with linear algebra that any number of layers can be reduced to the standard two-layer input-output model. What makes a multilayer perceptron different is that some neurons use a *nonlinear* activation function which was developed to model the frequency of action potentials, or firing, of biological neurons in the brain. This function is modeled in several ways.

The two main activation functions used in current applications are both sigmoids, and are described by

$$y(v_i) = \tanh(v_i) \text{ and } y(v_i) = (1 + e^{-v_i})^{-1},$$

in which the former function is a hyperbolic tangent which ranges from -1 to 1, and the latter, the logistic function, is similar in shape but ranges from 0 to 1. Here y_i is the output of the ith node (neuron) and v_i is the weighted sum of the input synapses. Alternative activation functions have been proposed, including the rectifier and softplus functions. More specialized activation functions include radial basis functions which are used in another class of supervised neural network models.

Layers

The multilayer perceptron consists of three or more layers (an input and an output layer with one or more *hidden layers*) of nonlinearly-activating nodes and is thus considered a deep neural network. Since an MLP is a Fully Connected Network, each node in one layer connects with a certain weight w_{ij} to every node in the following layer. Some people do not include the input layer when counting the number of layers and there is disagreement about whether w_{ij} should be interpreted as the weight from i to j or the other way around.

Learning Through Backpropagation

Learning occurs in the perceptron by changing connection weights after each piece of data is processed, based on the amount of error in the output compared to the expected result. This is an example of supervised learning, and is carried out through backpropagation, a generalization of the least mean squares algorithm in the linear perceptron.

We represent the error in output node j in the nth data point (training example) by

$e_j(n) = d_j(n) - y_j(n)$, where d is the target value and y is the value produced by the perceptron. We then make corrections to the weights of the nodes based on those corrections which minimize the error in the entire output, given by

$$\mathcal{E}(n) = \frac{1}{2} \sum_j e_j^2(n).$$

Using gradient descent, we find our change in each weight to be

$$\Delta w_{ji}(n) = -\eta \frac{\partial \mathcal{E}(n)}{\partial v_j(n)} y_i(n)$$

where y_i is the output of the previous neuron and η is the *learning rate*, which is carefully selected to ensure that the weights converge to a response fast enough, without producing oscillations.

The derivative to be calculated depends on the induced local field v_j, which itself varies. It is easy to prove that for an output node this derivative can be simplified to

$$-\frac{\partial \mathcal{E}(n)}{\partial v_j(n)} = e_j(n)\phi'(v_j(n))$$

where ϕ' is the derivative of the activation function described above, which itself does not vary. The analysis is more difficult for the change in weights to a hidden node, but it can be shown that the relevant derivative is

$$-\frac{\partial \mathcal{E}(n)}{\partial v_j(n)} = \phi'(v_j(n)) \sum_k -\frac{\partial \mathcal{E}(n)}{\partial v_k(n)} w_{kj}(n)$$

This depends on the change in weights of the kth nodes, which represent the output layer. So to change the hidden layer weights, we must first change the output layer weights according to the derivative of the activation function, and so this algorithm represents a *backpropagation of the activation function*.

Terminology

The term "multilayer perceptron" often causes confusion. It is argued the model is not a single perceptron that has multiple layers. Rather, it contains many perceptrons that are organised into layers, leading some to believe that a more fitting term might therefore be "multilayer perceptron network". Moreover, these "perceptrons" are not really perceptrons in the strictest possible sense, as true perceptrons are a special case of artificial neurons that use a threshold activation function such as the Heaviside step function, whereas the artificial neurons in a multilayer perceptron are free to take on any arbitrary activation function. Consequently, whereas a true perceptron performs binary classification, a neuron in a multilayer perceptron is free to either perform classification or regression, depending upon its activation function.

The two arguments raised above can be reconciled with the name "multilayer perceptron" if "perceptron" is simply interpreted to mean a binary classifier, independent of the specific mechanistic implementation of a classical perceptron. In this case, the entire network can indeed be considered to be a binary classifier with multiple layers. Furthermore, the term "multilayer perceptron" now does not specify the nature of the layers; the layers are free to be composed of general artificial neurons, and not perceptrons specifically. This interpretation of the term "multilayer perceptron" avoids the loosening of the definition of "perceptron" to mean an artificial neuron in general.

Applications

Multilayer perceptrons using a backpropagation algorithm are the standard algorithm for any supervised learning pattern recognition process and the subject of ongoing research in computational neuroscience and parallel distributed processing. They are useful in research in terms of their ability to solve problems stochastically, which often allows one to get approximate solutions for extremely complex problems like fitness approximation.

MLPs are universal function approximators as showed by Cybenko's theorem, so they can be used to create mathematical models by regression analysis. As classification is a particular case of regression when the response variable is categorical, MLPs are also good classifier algorithms.

MLPs were a popular machine learning solution in the 1980s, finding applications in diverse fields such as speech recognition, image recognition, and machine translation software, but have since the 1990s faced strong competition from the much simpler (and related) support vector machines. More recently, there has been some renewed interest in backpropagation networks due to the successes of deep learning.

Improvements over Perceptron:

1) Smooth nonlinearity - sigmoid

2) 1 or more hidden layers

Adding a Hidden Layer:

The perceptron, which has no hidden layers, can classify only linearly separable patterns. The MLP, with at least 1 hidden layer can classify *any* linearly non-separable classes also. An MLP can approximate any continuous multivariate function to any degree of accuracy, provided there are sufficiently many hidden neurons (Cybenko, 1988; Hornik et al, 1989). A more precise formulation is given below.

A serious limitation disappears suddenly by adding a single hidden layer.

It can easily be shown that the XOR problem which was not solvable by a Perceptron can be solved by a MLP with a single hidden layer containing two neurons.

XOR Example:

Neuron 1:

$$V_1 = \sigma(x_1 + x_2 - 1.5)$$

$$V_2 = \sigma(x_1 + x_2 - 0.5)$$

$$y = \sigma(V_1 - V_2 - 0.5)$$

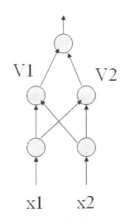

MLP for solving Xor

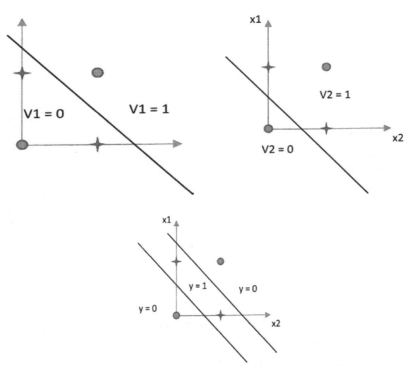

Plots showing the classification by V1,V2 and y(output of MLP)

Training the Hidden Layer

Not obvious how to train the hidden layer parameters.

The error term is meaningful only to the weights connected to the output layer. How to adjust hidden layer connections so as to reduce output error? – *credit assignment* problem.

Any connection can be adapted by taking a full partial derivative over the error function, but then to update a single weight in the first stage we need information about distant neurons/connections close to the output layer (locality rule is violated). In a large network with many layers, this implies that information is exchanged over distant elements of the network though they are not directly connected. Such an algorithm may be mathematically valid, but is biologically unrealistic.

References

- "CiteSeerX — Recurrent Multilayer Perceptrons for Identification and Control: The Road to Applications". Citeseerx.ist.psu.edu. Retrieved 2014-01-03

- Ganesan, N. "Application of Neural Networks in Diagnosing Cancer Disease Using Demographic Data" (PDF). International Journal of Computer Applications

- Minsky, M.; S. Papert (1969). Perceptrons: An Introduction to Computational Geometry. MIT Press. ISBN 0-262-63022-2

- Burgess, Matt. "DeepMind's AI learned to ride the London Underground using human-like reason and memory". WIRED UK. Retrieved 2016-10-19

- Salakhutdinov, Ruslan; Hinton, Geoffrey (2009). "Semantic hashing". International Journal of Approximate Reasoning. 50 (7): 969–978. doi:10.1016/j.ijar.2008.11.006

- Simonite, Tom. "Microsoft says its racist chatbot illustrates how AI isn't adaptable enough to help most businesses". MIT Technology Review. Retrieved 2017-04-10

- Russell, Stuart; Norvig, Peter (2003) [1995]. Artificial Intelligence: A Modern Approach (2nd ed.). Prentice Hall. ISBN 978-0137903955

- Mannes, John. "DeepMind's differentiable neural computer helps you navigate the subway with its memory". TechCrunch. Retrieved 2016-10-19

- Adrian, Edward D. (1926). "The impulses produced by sensory nerve endings". The Journal of Physiology. 61 (1): 49–72. doi:10.1113/jphysiol.1926.sp002273

- Mohri, Mehryar; Rostamizadeh, Afshin; Talwalkar, Ameet (2012). Foundations of Machine Learning. USA, Massachusetts: MIT Press. ISBN 9780262018258

- Balcázar, José (Jul 1997). "Computational Power of Neural Networks: A Kolmogorov Complexity Characterization". Information Theory, IEEE Transactions on. 43 (4): 1175–1183. doi:10.1109/18.605580. Retrieved 3 November 2014

- Felix Gers, Nicholas Schraudolph, and Jürgen Schmidhuber (2002). Learning precise timing with LSTM recurrent networks. Journal of Machine Learning Research 3:115–143

- Alpaydin, Ethem (2010). Introduction to Machine Learning. London: The MIT Press. ISBN 978-0-262-01243-0. Retrieved 4 February 2017

- C.W. Omlin, C.L. Giles, "Constructing Deterministic Finite-State Automata in Recurrent Neural Networks" Journal of the ACM, 45(6), 937-972, 1996

- Cornell University Library. "Breiman : Statistical Modeling: The Two Cultures (with comments and a rejoinder by the author)". Retrieved 8 August 2015

- Bishop, Christopher M. "Chapter 4. Linear Models for Classification". Pattern Recognition and Machine Learning. Springer Science+Business Media, LLC. p. 194. ISBN 978-0387-31073-2

- "With QuickType, Apple wants to do more than guess your next text. It wants to give you an AI.". WIRED. Retrieved 2016-06-16

- F. Gomez, J. Schmidhuber, R. Miikkulainen. Accelerated Neural Evolution through Cooperatively Coevolved Synapses. Journal of Machine Learning Research (JMLR), 9:937-965, 2008

Unsupervised Learning: An Integrated Study

Unsupervised machine learning ascertains a function to find the hidden data from unlabeled data as opposed to supervised machine learning, which conducts the same operation from labeled data. The section explores the concept of Hebbian theory, which is one of the major approaches taken by unsupervised machine learning. It comes up with an explanation to the adaption of neurons during the learning process. The major forms of unsupervised machine learning are dealt with great details in the section.

Unsupervised Learning

Unsupervised machine learning is the machine learning task of inferring a function to describe hidden structure from "unlabeled" data (a classification or categorization is not included in the observations). Since the examples given to the learner are unlabeled, there is no evaluation of the accuracy of the structure that is output by the relevant algorithm—which is one way of distinguishing unsupervised learning from supervised learning and reinforcement learning.

A central case of unsupervised learning is the problem of density estimation in statistics, though unsupervised learning encompasses many other problems (and solutions) involving summarizing and explaining key features of the data.

Approaches to unsupervised learning include:

- clustering
    - k-means
    - mixture models
    - hierarchical clustering,
- anomaly detection
- Neural Networks
    - Hebbian Learning
    - Generative Adversarial Networks
- Approaches for learning latent variable models such as
    - Expectation–maximization algorithm (EM)
    - Method of moments

    o   Blind signal separation techniques, e.g.,

- Principal component analysis,

- Independent component analysis,

- Non-negative matrix factorization,

- Singular value decomposition.

Unsupervised Learning in Neural Networks

The classical example of unsupervised learning in the study of both natural and artificial neural networks is subsumed by Donald Hebb's principle, that is, neurons that fire together wire together. In Hebbian learning, the connection is reinforced irrespective of an error, but is exclusively a function of the coincidence between action potentials between the two neurons. A similar version that modifies synaptic weights takes into account the time between the action potentials (spike-timing-dependent plasticity or STDP). Hebbian Learning has been hypothesized to underlie a range of cognitive functions, such as pattern recognition and experiential learning.

Among neural network models, the self-organizing map (SOM) and adaptive resonance theory (ART) are commonly used unsupervised learning algorithms. The SOM is a topographic organization in which nearby locations in the map represent inputs with similar properties. The ART model allows the number of clusters to vary with problem size and lets the user control the degree of similarity between members of the same clusters by means of a user-defined constant called the vigilance parameter. ART networks are also used for many pattern recognition tasks, such as automatic target recognition and seismic signal processing. The first version of ART was "ART1", developed by Carpenter and Grossberg (1988).

Method of Moments

One of the statistical approaches for unsupervised learning is the method of moments. In the method of moments, the unknown parameters (of interest) in the model are related to the moments of one or more random variables, and thus, these unknown parameters can be estimated given the moments. The moments are usually estimated from samples empirically. The basic moments are first and second order moments. For a random vector, the first order moment is the mean vector, and the second order moment is the covariance matrix (when the mean is zero). Higher order moments are usually represented using tensors which are the generalization of matrices to higher orders as multi-dimensional arrays.

In particular, the method of moments is shown to be effective in learning the parameters of latent variable models. Latent variable models are statistical models where in addition to the observed variables, a set of latent variables also exists which is not observed. A highly practical example of latent variable models in machine learning is the topic modeling which is a statistical model for generating the words (observed variables) in the document based on the topic (latent variable) of the document. In the topic modeling, the words in the document are generated according to different statistical parameters when the topic of the document is changed. It is shown that method of moments (tensor decomposition techniques) consistently recover the parameters of a large class of latent variable models under some assumptions.

The Expectation–maximization algorithm (EM) is also one of the most practical methods for learning latent variable models. However, it can get stuck in local optima, and it is not guaranteed that the algorithm will converge to the true unknown parameters of the model. Alternatively, for the method of moments, the global convergence is guaranteed under some conditions.

Examples

Behavioral-based detection in network security has become a good application area for a combination of supervised- and unsupervised-machine learning. This is because the amount of data for a human security analyst to analyze is impossible (measured in terabytes per day) to review to find patterns and anomalies. According to Giora Engel, co-founder of LightCyber, in a *Dark Reading* article, "The great promise machine learning holds for the security industry is its ability to detect advanced and unknown attacks -- particularly those leading to data breaches." The basic premise is that a motivated attacker will find their way into a network (generally by compromising a user's computer or network account through phishing, social engineering or malware). The security challenge then becomes finding the attacker by their operational activities, which include reconnaissance, lateral movement, command & control and exfiltration. These activities--especially reconnaissance and lateral movement--stand in contrast to an established baseline of "normal" or "good" activity for each user and device on the network. The role of machine learning is to create ongoing profiles for users and devices and then find meaningful anomalies.

Hebbian Theory

Hebbian theory is a theory in neuroscience that proposes an explanation for the adaptation of neurons in the brain during the learning process, describing a basic mechanism for synaptic plasticity, where an increase in synaptic efficacy arises from the presynaptic cell's repeated and persistent stimulation of the postsynaptic cell. Introduced by Donald Hebb in his 1949 book *The Organization of Behavior*, the theory is also called Hebb's rule, Hebb's postulate, and cell assembly theory. Hebb states it as follows:

Let us assume that the persistence or repetition of a reverberatory activity (or "trace") tends to induce lasting cellular changes that add to its stability.[...] When an axon of cell *A* is near enough to excite a cell *B* and repeatedly or persistently takes part in firing it, some growth process or metabolic change takes place in one or both cells such that *A*'s efficiency, as one of the cells firing *B*, is increased.

The theory is often summarized by Siegrid Löwel's phrase: "Cells that fire together, wire together." However, this summary should not be taken literally. Hebb emphasized that cell A needs to "take part in firing" cell B, and such causality can only occur if cell A fires just before, not at the same time as, cell B. This important aspect of causation in Hebb's work foreshadowed what is now known about spike-timing-dependent plasticity, which requires temporal precedence. The theory attempts to explain associative or Hebbian learning, in which simultaneous activation of cells leads to pronounced increases in synaptic strength between those cells, and provides a biological basis for errorless learning methods for education and memory rehabilitation. In the study of neural networks in cognitive function, it is often regarded as the neuronal basis of unsupervised learning.

Hebbian Engrams and Cell Assembly Theory

Hebbian theory concerns how neurons might connect themselves to become engrams. Hebb's theories on the form and function of cell assemblies can be understood from the following: "The general idea is an old one, that any two cells or systems of cells that are repeatedly active at the same time will tend to become 'associated', so that activity in one facilitates activity in the other." He also wrote: "When one cell repeatedly assists in firing another, the axon of the first cell develops synaptic knobs (or enlarges them if they already exist) in contact with the soma of the second cell."

Gordon Allport posits additional ideas regarding cell assembly theory and its role in forming engrams, along the lines of the concept of auto-association, described as follows:

If the inputs to a system cause the same pattern of activity to occur repeatedly, the set of active elements constituting that pattern will become increasingly strongly interassociated. That is, each element will tend to turn on every other element and (with negative weights) to turn off the elements that do not form part of the pattern. To put it another way, the pattern as a whole will become 'auto-associated'. We may call a learned (auto-associated) pattern an engram.

Hebbian theory has been the primary basis for the conventional view that, when analyzed from a holistic level, engrams are neuronal nets or neural networks.

Work in the laboratory of Eric Kandel has provided evidence for the involvement of Hebbian learning mechanisms at synapses in the marine gastropod *Aplysia californica*.

Experiments on Hebbian synapse modification mechanisms at the central nervous system synapses of vertebrates are much more difficult to control than are experiments with the relatively simple peripheral nervous system synapses studied in marine invertebrates. Much of the work on long-lasting synaptic changes between vertebrate neurons (such as long-term potentiation) involves the use of non-physiological experimental stimulation of brain cells. However, some of the physiologically relevant synapse modification mechanisms that have been studied in vertebrate brains do seem to be examples of Hebbian processes. One such study reviews results from experiments that indicate that long-lasting changes in synaptic strengths can be induced by physiologically relevant synaptic activity working through both Hebbian and non-Hebbian mechanisms.

Principles

From the point of view of artificial neurons and artificial neural networks, Hebb's principle can be described as a method of determining how to alter the weights between model neurons. The weight between two neurons increases if the two neurons activate simultaneously, and reduces if they activate separately. Nodes that tend to be either both positive or both negative at the same time have strong positive weights, while those that tend to be opposite have strong negative weights.

The following is a formulaic description of Hebbian learning: (note that many other descriptions are possible)

$$w_{ij} = x_i x_j$$

where w_{ij} is the weight of the connection from neuron j to neuron i and x_i the input for neuron i. Note that this is pattern learning (weights updated after every training example). In a Hopfield network, connections w_{ij} are set to zero if $i = j$ (no reflexive connections allowed). With binary neurons (activations either 0 or 1), connections would be set to 1 if the connected neurons have the same activation for a pattern.

Another formulaic description is:

$$w_{ij} = \frac{1}{p} \sum_{k=1}^{p} x_i^k x_j^k,$$

where w_{ij} is the weight of the connection from neuron j to neuron i, p is the number of training patterns, and x_i^k the kth input for neuron i. This is learning by epoch (weights updated after all the training examples are presented). Again, in a Hopfield network, connections $_{ij}$ are set to zero if $i = j$ (no reflexive connections).

A variation of Hebbian learning that takes into account phenomena such as blocking and many other neural learning phenomena is the mathematical model of Harry Klopf. Klopf's model reproduces a great many biological phenomena, and is also simple to implement.

Generalization and Stability

Hebb's Rule is often generalized as

$$\Delta w_i = \eta x_i y,$$

or the change in the ith synaptic weight w_i is equal to a learning rate η times the ith input x_i times the postsynaptic response y. Often cited is the case of a linear neuron,

$$y = \sum_j w_j x_j,$$

and the simplification takes both the learning rate and the input weights to be 1. This version of the rule is clearly unstable, as in any network with a dominant signal the synaptic weights will increase or decrease exponentially. However, it can be shown that for *any* neuron model, Hebb's rule is unstable. Therefore, network models of neurons usually employ other learning theories such as BCM theory, Oja's rule, or the Generalized Hebbian Algorithm.

Exceptions

Despite the common use of Hebbian models for long-term potentiation, there exist several exceptions to Hebb's principles and examples that demonstrate that some aspects of the theory are oversimplified. One of the most well-documented of these exceptions pertains to how synaptic modification may not simply occur only between activated neurons A and B, but to neighboring neurons as well. This is due to how Hebbian modification depends on retrograde signaling in order to modify the presynaptic neuron. The compound most commonly identified as fulfilling this retrograde transmitter role is nitric oxide, which, due to its high solubility and diffusibility, often exerts effects on nearby neurons. This type of diffuse synaptic modification, known as volume learning, counters, or at least supplements, the traditional Hebbian model.

Hebbian Learning Account of Mirror Neurons

Hebbian learning and spike-timing-dependent plasticity have been used in an influential theory of how mirror neurons emerge. Mirror neurons are neurons that fire both when an individual performs an action and when the individual sees or hears another perform a similar action. The discovery of these neurons has been very influential in explaining how individuals make sense of the actions of others, by showing that, when a person perceives the actions of others, the person activates the motor programs which they would use to perform similar actions. The activation of these motor programs then adds information to the perception and helps predict what the person will do next based on the perceiver's own motor program. A challenge has been to explain how individuals come to have neurons that respond both while performing an action and while hearing or seeing another perform similar actions.

Christian Keysers and David Perrett suggested that, while an individual performs a particular action, the individual will see, hear, and feel himself perform the action. These re-afferent sensory signals will trigger activity in neurons responding to the sight, sound, and feel of the action. Because the activity of these sensory neurons will consistently overlap in time with those of the motor neurons that caused the action, Hebbian learning would predict that the synapses connecting neurons responding to the sight, sound, and feel of an action and those of the neurons triggering the action should be potentiated. The same is true while people look at themselves in the mirror, hear themselves babble, or are imitated by others. After repeated experience of this re-afference, the synapses connecting the sensory and motor representations of an action would be so strong that the motor neurons would start firing to the sound or the vision of the action, and a mirror neuron would have been created.

Evidence for that perspective comes from many experiments that show that motor programs can be triggered by novel auditory or visual stimuli after repeated pairing of the stimulus with the execution of the motor program. For instance, people who have never played the piano do not activate brain regions involved in playing the piano when listening to piano music. Five hours of piano lessons, in which the participant is exposed to the sound of the piano each time he presses a key, suffices to later trigger activity in motor regions of the brain upon listening to piano music. Consistent with the fact that spike-timing-dependent plasticity occurs only if the presynaptic neuron's firing predicts the post-synaptic neuron's firing, the link between sensory stimuli and motor programs also only seem to be potentiated if the stimulus is contingent on the motor program.

Linear Neuron Model: (Hebbian Learning)

$$y = \sum_{i=1}^{n} w_i x_i$$

In vector form:

$$y = w \bullet x$$

Apply Hebbian learning,

$$\Delta w_i = \eta y x_i$$

$$\Delta w = \eta y x$$

$$= \eta(w^{T}x)x = \eta x(x^{T}w) = \eta(xx^{T})w$$

For multiple patterns the learning rule is,

$$\Delta w = \eta \sum_{p}(x(p)x(p)^{T})w$$

$$R = \sum_{p}x(p)x(p)^{T}$$

R is the autocorrelation matrix of training data. It is:

-   symmetric,

-   positive semi-definite

Proof:

1) Symmetric:

$$R_{ij} = \sum_{p}x_{i}(p)x_{j}(p) = R_{ji}$$

2) Positive semi-definite:

Consider the quadratic form associated with R,

$$\frac{1}{2}u^{T}Ru,$$

where u is a non-zero real vector.

$$\frac{1}{2}u^{T}Ru = \frac{1}{2}u^{T}(\sum_{p}x(p)x(p)^{T})u$$

$$= \frac{1}{2}(\sum_{p}(u^{T}x(p))(x(p)^{T}u))$$

$$= \frac{1}{2}\sum_{p}(u^{T}x(p))^{2} \geq 0$$

$$\Delta w = \eta Rw$$

In differential equation form,

$$\dot{w} = Rw$$

•   Maximize $\frac{1}{2}w^{T}Rw$

Therefore, hebbian learning of a linear neuron

•   Maximizing the quadratic form, E, of R

$$E(w) = \frac{1}{2}w^{T}Rw$$

$$= \frac{1}{2}(\sum_p (w^T x(p))(x(p)^T w))$$

$$= \frac{1}{2}(\sum_p (w^T x(p))^2 = \frac{1}{2}\sum_p (y(p))^2$$

Therefore, Hebbian learning of a linear neuron

- Maximizing the quadratic form of $R\left(=\frac{1}{2}w^T R w\right)$

- Maximizing the average squared output of the neuron.

- We also note that if the data is 'zero mean' ($E[x] = 0$), Hebbian learning also maximizes output variance. Since the neuron is linear, for zero-mean input data, mean squared value of the output equals output variance. i.e.,

$$E\left[y^2\right] = \sigma_y^2$$

But if R is positive semi-definite, E (w) does not have a maximum. Therefore, E must be constrained. A simple constraint is to make w a unit norm vector. The unit norm constraint can be added as a cost to E(w), yielding the new E' as follows:

$$E(w) = \frac{1}{2}w^T R w - \frac{1}{2}\lambda(\|w\|^2 - 1)$$

Here, λ is the Lagragian multiplier.

Calculating the gradient,

$$\nabla_w E(w) = Rw - \lambda w = 0,$$

or

$$Rw - \lambda w$$

which is an eigenvalue equation

Therefore, when trained by Hebbian learning, the weight vector of a linear neuron converges to the eigenvectors of the autocorrelation matrix, R.

But since a symmetric real matrix of size 'n Xn' has n eigenvectors, it is not clear which of them w tends to.

We will show that w tends to the eigenvector corresponding to the highest eigenvalue.

Proof:

Let Q be a orthogonal, diagonalizing matrix Q such that,

$$Q^T R Q = \wedge$$

Where

$$\wedge = \begin{bmatrix} \lambda_1 & 0 & 0 \\ 0 & \lambda_1 & 0 \\ 0 & 0 & \lambda_n \end{bmatrix}$$

$$Q = [q_1 | \ldots | q_i | \ldots | q_n]$$

Where q_i are the eigenvectors of R.

Now consider the linear transformation,

$$w = Qx,$$

and express E(w) in terms of x, as follows,

$$E(w) = \frac{1}{2}(Qx)^T RQx$$

$$= \frac{1}{2}x^T Q^T RQx = \frac{1}{2}x^T \wedge x = \frac{1}{2}\sum_{i=1}^{n}\lambda_i x_i^2$$

Since Q is also a rotational transformation, maximum of the new function E(x) is the same as the maximum of the older function E(w). Let us consider the maximum of E'(x),

Let the eigenvalues of R be ordered such that,

$$\lambda_1 \geq \ldots \geq \lambda_i \geq \ldots \lambda_n$$

$$E(x) = \frac{1}{2}\sum_{i=1}^{n}\lambda_i x_i^2$$

We now impose the unit norm constraint on x as follows,

$$\frac{1}{2}\sum_{i=1}^{n}(\lambda_i x_i^2)$$

$$\frac{1}{2}(\lambda_1(1 - \sum_{i \neq 1}x_i^2) + \sum_{i \neq 1}^{n}\lambda_i x_i^2)$$

The maximum of the above function can be found by solving the following differential equations,

$$\frac{dx_i}{dt} = (\lambda_i - \lambda_1)x_i$$

There are (n-1) such equations corresponding to (n-1) components, x_i i = 2,...n.

Since λ_1 is the largest eigenvalue, in all the above differential equations, $x_i \to 0$, i = 2,...n.

Since $\|x\| = 1$, the only remaining component $x_1 = 1$. Therefore the maximum of E(x) occurs when, $x = [1\ 0\ 0...0]$.

Since w = Qx, we have, w = q_1.

Thus the weight vector of the linear neuron of eqn. converges to the eigenvector corresponding to the highest eigenvalue of E, when trained by Hebbian learning.

Oja's Rule

Under the action of Hebbian learning, weight vector of a linear neuron converged to the first eigenvector of R only when the weights are normalized as $\|w\| = 1$.

But such a condition is artificial and not part of the Hebbian mechanism which is biologically motivated. Therefore, Oja (1982) proposed a modification of Hebbian mechanism in which the weight vector is automatically normalized without explicitly an explicit step like,

$$w \rightarrow w / \|w\|$$

The weight update according to Oja (1982) is as follows:

$$\Delta w_i = \eta y(x_i - y w_i)$$

In vector form, the update rule can be written as,

$$\Delta w = \eta y(x - yw)$$

Let us prove that the above rule does the following:

- Maximizes $\frac{1}{2} w^T R w$

- $\|w\| = 1$

Consider the average update in w for the entire data set S, when the weight vector converges

$$E[\Delta w] = \eta E[y(x - yw)] = 0$$

$$= \eta E[(yx - y^2 w)]$$

$$= \eta E[((w^T x)x - (w^T x)^2 w)]$$

$$= \eta[(E(xx^T)w - E(w^T (xx^T)w)w)]$$

$$= \eta[(Rw - (w^T Rw)w)] = 0$$

The last equation is the eigenvalue equation in R.

$$Rw - \lambda w = 0$$

Thus w is an eigenvector of R.

where $\lambda = w^T R w$

or $\lambda = w^T (\lambda w)$

$\Rightarrow \|w\| = 1$

Like Hebbian learning, an advantage of Oja's rule is that it is local: update for the i'th component,- w_i, of the weight vector, w, is dependent on quantities that are locally available at the presynaptic or postsynaptic ends of the synapse that is represented by w_i.

Example:

Long term potentiation in hippocampal neurons of brain

Principal Component Analysis and Hebbian Learning

Before we proceed to prove an interesting result relating Hebbian learning and principal component analysis (PCA) we state a result from linear algebra.

Spectral Theorem: If R is a real symmetric matrix, and Q is an orthogonal, diagonalizingmatrix such that,

$$Q^T RQ = \wedge$$

Where

$$\wedge = \begin{bmatrix} \lambda_1 & 0 & 0 \\ 0 & \lambda_i & 0 \\ 0 & 0 & \lambda_n \end{bmatrix} Q = \begin{bmatrix} q1 | ... | qi | ... | qn \end{bmatrix}$$

Then

$$R = \sum_{i=1}^{n} \lambda_i q_i q_i^T$$

Proof:

Since,

$$Q^T RQ = \wedge$$

$$R = Q \wedge_{Q^T}$$

$$= \sum_{i=1}^{n} \lambda_i q_i q_i^T$$

To derive the last result, we used the following,

$$q_i q_j^T = \delta(i,j)$$

Where $\delta(i,j)$ is the Kronecker delta, defined as,

$$\delta(i,j) = 1, \quad \text{if} (i = j)$$

$= 1$, otherwise

We have shown earlier that, Hebbian learning of a linear neuron

- Maximizing the quadratic form of $R = \left(= \frac{1}{2} w^T R w \right)$

- Maximizing the average squared output of the neuron.

- We also note that if the data is 'zero mean' ($E[x] = 0$), Hebbian learning also maximizes output variance.Since the neuron is linear, for zero-mean input data, mean squared value of the output equals output variance. i.e.,

$$E[y]^2 = \sigma_y^2$$

We now show that Hebbian learning can used for data compression. Using this mechanism, a vector, x, of dimension, n, can transformed into another vector, y, of dimension, m, (m <n), such that x can be reconstructed from y, with minimum reconstruction error.

To enable such compression, we assume, for the moment, the following:

We have seen that Hebbian learning extracts the eigenvector corresponding to the largest eigenvalue of the autocorrelation matrix, R. But we assume that it is possible to extract all the eigenvectors of R, by some sort of an extension of Hebbian learning. But for now we assume such an extension, and describe how data compression can be achieved by Hebbian learning.

Let x, be a data point drawn from a data set S. R is the autocorrelation matrix associated with S. Assume that the data is zero-mean ($E[x]=0$). Q is a matrix constructed out of the eigenvectors of R as follows,

$$Q = \left[q_1 | \cdots | q_i | \cdots | q_n \right]$$

Consider the following linear transformation,

$$y = Q^T x$$

Note that the components of y, are the projections of x onto the first m eigenvectors of R.

$$y_i = q_i^T x$$

Let us calculate the variance of y_i, which we will use shortly.

Since the data set, S, is zero-mean,

$E[x] = 0$. Therefore, from linearity of eqn. above, we have $E[yi]=0$. Therefore,

$$\sigma_{y_i}^2 = E\left[y_i^2 \right] = E\left[\left(q_i^T x \right) \left(q_i^T x \right) \right]$$
$$= q_i^T E\left[x^T x \right] q_i$$
$$= q_i^T R q_i = q_i^T \lambda_i q_i = \lambda_i$$

Thus the variance of the i'th component,y_i , is the corresponding eigenvalue.

'x' can be reconstructed from y, by simply inverting the transformation of eqn.

$$x = Qy$$

In the last equation, x can be expressed as a weighted sum eigenvectors as,

$$x = \sum_{i=1}^{n} q_i\, y_i$$

Eigenvectors are ordered such that the corresponding eigenvalues are in the descending order.

$$\lambda_1 \geq \dots \geq \lambda_i \geq \dots \lambda_n$$

Now consider a reconstruction of x, denoted by $\tilde{x}$, produced by taking only a partial summation of the expression in eqn. above.

$$\hat{x} = \sum_{i=1}^{m} q_i y_i$$

Reconstruction error,

$$e = x - \tilde{x} = \sum_{i=1}^{n} q_i y_i - \sum_{i=1}^{m} q_i y_i = \sum_{i=m+1}^{n} q_i y_i$$

Root Mean Square (RMS) value of the reconstruction error is,

$$E\left[e\, e\right] \quad E\left[\left(\sum_{i=m+1}^{n} q_i y_i\right)\left(\sum_{i=m+1}^{n} q_i y_i\right)\right]$$

$$= E\left[\left(\sum_{i=m+1}^{n} q\ q_i y_i^2\right)\right] = E\left[\left(\sum_{i=m+1}^{n} y_i^2\right)\right] =$$

$$= \sum_{i=m+1}^{n} E\left[y_i\right] = \sum_{i=m+1}^{n} {}_i$$

Thus the reconstruction error is the sum of lower (corresponding to larger i) eigenvalues of R. As m increases, and approaches n, error reduces since there are fewer terms in the expansion of eqn. But error decreases also because the eigenvalues are sorted and lower eigenvalues are smaller in magnitude than higher ones (larger i).

Typically, in high-dimensional real-world data, there are a small number of large-valued eigenvalues, and a large number of small-valued eigenvalues. If 'm' is chosen such that the larger eigenvalues are included, x can be expressed in a compressed form, y, and reconstructed again, $\hat{x}$ ",with minimal loss.

Example:

1. Take random 100 dim data. Show the distribution of eigenvalues.

Taken a random 100 dim data distributed between 0 and 1. The Eigen value is distributed as Figure.

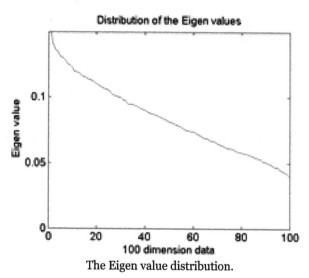

The Eigen value distribution.

Code:

```
%consider an artificial data set of 100 variables (e.g., genes) and 10
samples
data=rand(100,1000);
% remove the mean variable-wise (row-wise)
data=data-repmat(mean(data,2),1,size(data,2));
% calculate eigenvectors (loadings) W, and eigenvalues of the covariance
matrix
[W, EvalueMatrix] = eig(cov(data'));
Evalues = diag(EvalueMatrix);
% order by largest eigenvalue
Evalues = Evalues(end:-1:1);
%Plotting
figure(1);set(gca,'FontSize',14)
plot(Evalues);
ylim([0 .15]);
ylabel('Eigen value');
```

```
xlabel('100 dimension data');

title('Distribution of the Eigen values');
```

Sanger's Rule

We have seen that Hebb's rule gives the weight vector that is the first eigenvector of the autocorrelation matrix R. Oja's rule also essentially provided the same result, with the distinction that it achieved normalization naturally. It would be desirable to extend these results to the case of m-principal components. Two such extensions are available – one due to Sanger (1989) and the other due again to Oja (1989).

Since M-principal components need to be discovered in this case, we have a network with 'm' output neurons. The neurons are linear as before. The output of the i'th output neuron can therefore be expressed as,

$$y_i = \sum_{i=1}^{m} w_{ij} x_j$$

The above equation in matrix form becomes,

$$y = w_i^T x = x^T w_i$$

The weights are trained by the following rule (Sanger, 1989):

$$\Delta w_{ij} = \eta y_i \left(x_i - \sum_{k=1}^{i} w_{kj} x_k \right)$$

Linsker's Model

Ralf Linsker proposed a model of the visual system that consists of a multilayered network trained by Hebbian learning. The layers in the network are two-dimensional, analogous to the sheets of neurons in various stages of the real visual system. Neurons are all layers are linear. Each neuron in a given layer receives inputs from a local neighborhood in the previous layers, a feature that is also inspired the connectivity patterns in the visual system. Since all the neurons are linear, the entire network has linear input-output relationship. Therefore, it may not be capable of representing rich input-output characteristics, and does not enjoy the universal approximation property of the MLPs. But the training is done is stages, one layer at a time. Due to such layer-wise training, weights in each weight stage evolve differently, producing interesting response patterns like orientation sensitivity, exhibited by neurons in the primary visual cortex.

Consider the response, y, of a neuron in one of the layers of Linsker's model.

$$y = a + \sum_{j=1}^{K} w_j V_j$$

V_j could be the input pattern, x_j, or the response of a neuron in the previous layer.

A variation of Hebb's rule is used to train the weights, w_i:

$$\Delta w_i = \eta\left(V_i y + b V_i + c y + d\right)$$

The first term on the right-hand side (the product $V_i y$) is the product term that appears in the original Hebb's rule. The remaining terms are linear and constant terms that appear in Linsker's variation.

The parameters b, c and d can be tuned appropriately so that neurons in various layers display various response properties. The weights are prevented from blowing up by clipping them as follows,

$$w_- < w_i < w_+$$

To compute the final values to which the weights converge, let us consider the average change in weights, which must be zero at convergence.

$$0 = E\left[\Delta w_i\right] = \eta(E\left[V_i y\right] + b E\left[V_i\right] + c E\left[y\right] + d)$$

Let $V_i = \bar{V} + v_i$, where $\bar{V} = E[V_i]$ and v_i is the deviation from the mean. Then,

$$E[\Delta w_i] = \eta(E\left[\left(\bar{V}+v_i\right)\left(a+\sum_j^K w_j\left(\bar{V}+v_j\right)\right)\right]+b\bar{V}+cE\left[\left(a+\sum_j^K w_j\left(\bar{V}+v_j\right)\right)\right]+d)$$

$$= \eta(aE\left[\left(\bar{V}+v_i\right)+E\left[\sum_j^K w_j\left(\bar{V}+v_j\right)\left(\bar{V}+v_i\right)\right]+b\bar{V}+ac+cE\left[\sum_j^K w_j\left(\bar{V}+v_j\right)\right]+d)\right.$$

$$= \eta(a\bar{V}+\sum_j^K w_j\,\bar{V}^2+E\left[\sum_j^K w_j v_j v_i\right]+b\bar{V}+ac+cE\left[\sum_j^K w_j\left(\bar{V}+v_j\right)\right]+d)$$

$$= \eta(a\bar{V}+\sum_j^K w_j\,\bar{V}^2+\sum_j^K w_j C_{ij}+b\bar{V}+ac+c\sum_j^K w_j\,\bar{V}+d)$$

Where Cij is the the (i,j) element of the covariance matrix $E[v_i v_j]$.

Terms in the last equation can be regrouped as,

$$= \eta(\sum_j^K w_j\,\bar{V}^2+\sum_j^K w_j C_{ij}+a\bar{V}+b\bar{V}+ac+d+c\sum_j^K w_j\,\bar{V}+d)$$

$$= \eta((\sum_j^K w_j C_{ij})+(a\bar{V}+b\bar{V}+ac+d)+(\bar{V}^2+c\bar{V})(\sum_j^K w_j))$$

$$= \eta((\sum_j^K w_j C_{ij})+\lambda(\mu-\sum_j^K w_j))$$

where λ and μ are functions of the constants a, b, c, d and $\bar{V}$.

The above weight dynamics can be interpreted as gradient descent over a cost function:

$$\Delta w_i = -\eta\frac{\partial E}{\partial w_i}$$

$$E = -\frac{1}{2}w^T C w + \frac{\lambda}{2}\left(\mu-\sum_j w_j\right)^2$$

The first term is similar to standard Hebbian learning that maximizes quadratic form associated with the autocorrelation matrix of the input data. The second term is a Lagrangian multiplier that imposes the condition

$$\sum_j w_j = \mu$$

on the weights.

Training Results

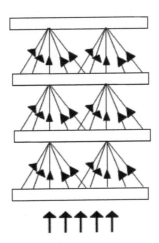

The Linsker's model (Layers A to G)

Linsker's model consist of 7 two-dimensional layers of neurons, A to G, where each layer projects to the subsequent layer in a 'pyramidal' fashion. Training is done in a sequential fashion. Weights of a stage are first trained to saturation, before the next stage is trained. Note that all training in this model is unsupervised governed by eqns. There is no attempt to map the input to some pre-specified target output.

Independent random noise is given as input to the first layer, A. therefore the autocorrelation matrix is an identity matrix. It was found that for a range of parameters all the weight saturated to w+. Since all the weights are the same, the response of Layer B is simply a local average, or smoothed version of the image presented to layer A. Therefore, neural activation in layer B turned out to have high local correlation. But beyond a small radius of high correlation, layer B neurons had low correlation.

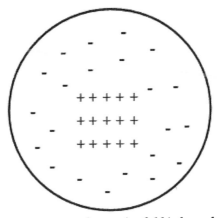

The Center-Surround receptive field in lower layers

Due to this reason, neurons in layer C developed center-surround kind of receptive fields. They responded strongly either to a bright dot with a dark background, or to a black dot with a white background. This trend continued to all the way to layer F where neurons had center-surround receptive fields.

But in Layer G the parameter values were changed. Therefore, trained produced a variety of weight patterns, many of them were asymmetric. Some neurons had receptive fields with alternating bands of positive and negative weights. Such cells had orientation sensitivity. Some other cells had a central positive region surrounding by several islands of negative regions.

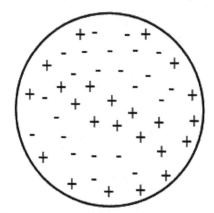

The orientation sensitivity in higher layers

Thus Linsker's model shows that in a multilayer model, trained by simple Hebbian mechanism, neurons in the lower layers had center-surround kind of receptive fields, while those of higher layers had orientation sensitivity.

Competitive Learning

Competitive learning is a form of unsupervised learning in artificial neural networks, in which nodes compete for the right to respond to a subset of the input data. A variant of Hebbian learning, competitive learning works by increasing the specialization of each node in the network. It is well suited to finding clusters within data.

Models and algorithms based on the principle of competitive learning include vector quantization and self-organizing maps (Kohonen maps).

Principles

There are three basic elements to a competitive learning rule:

- A set of neurons that are all the same except for some randomly distributed synaptic weights, and which therefore respond differently to a given set of input patterns

- A limit imposed on the "strength" of each neuron

- A mechanism that permits the neurons to compete for the right to respond to a given subset of inputs, such that only one output neuron (or only one neuron per group), is active (i.e. "on") at a time. The neuron that wins the competition is called a "winner-take-all" neuron.

Accordingly, the individual neurons of the network learn to specialize on ensembles of similar patterns and in so doing become 'feature detectors' for different classes of input patterns.

The fact that competitive networks recode sets of correlated inputs to one of a few output neurons essentially removes the redundancy in representation which is an essential part of processing in biological sensory systems.

Architecture and Implementation

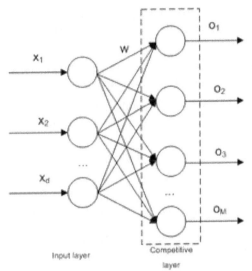

Competitive neural network architecture

Competitive Learning is usually implemented with Neural Networks that contain a hidden layer which is commonly known as "competitive layer". Every competitive neuron is described by a vector of weights $w_i = (w_{i1},..,w_{id})^T, i = 1,..,M$ and calculates the similarity measure between the input data $x^n = (x_{n1},..,x_{nd})^T \in \mathbb{R}^d$ and the weight vector w_i.

For every input vector, the competitive neurons "compete" with each other to see which one of them is the most similar to that particular input vector. The winner neuron m sets its output $o_m = 1$ and all the other competitive neurons set their output $o_i = 0, i = 1,..,M, i \neq m$.

Usually, in order to measure similarity the inverse of the Euclidean distance is used: $\|x - w_i\|$ between the input vector x^n and the weight vector w_i.

Example Algorithm

Here is a simple competitive learning algorithm to find three clusters within some input data.

1. (Set-up.) Let a set of sensors all feed into three different nodes, so that every node is connected to every sensor. Let the weights that each node gives to its sensors be set randomly between 0.0 and 1.0. Let the output of each node be the sum of all its sensors, each sensor's signal strength being multiplied by its weight.

2. When the net is shown an input, the node with the highest output is deemed the winner. The input is classified as being within the cluster corresponding to that node.

3. The winner updates each of its weights, moving weight from the connections that gave it weaker signals to the connections that gave it stronger signals.

Thus, as more data are received, each node converges on the centre of the cluster that it has come to represent and activates more strongly for inputs in this cluster and more weakly for inputs in other clusters.

References

- Euliano, Neil R. (1999-12-21). "Neural and Adaptive Systems: Fundamentals Through Simulations" (PDF). Neural and Adaptive Systems: Fundamentals Through Simulations. Wiley. Archived from the original (PDF) on 2015-12-25. Retrieved 2016-03-16

- Caporale N; Dan Y (2008). "Spike timing-dependent plasticity: a Hebbian learning rule". Annual Review of Neuroscience. 31: 25–46. PMID 18275283. doi:10.1146/annurev.neuro.31.060407.125639

- Allport, D.A. (1985). "Distributed memory, modular systems and dysphasia". In Newman, S.K.; Epstein R. (Eds.). Current Perspectives in Dysphasia. Edinburgh: Churchill Livingstone. ISBN 0-443-03039-1

- Shouval, Harel (2005-01-03). "The Physics of the Brain". The Synaptic basis for Learning and Memory: A theoretical approach. The University of Texas Health Science Center at Houston. Archived from the original on 2007-06-10. Retrieved 2007-11-14

- Mitchison, G; N. Swindale (October 1999). "Can Hebbian Volume Learning Explain Discontinuities in Cortical Maps?". Neural Computation. 11: 1519–1526. doi:10.1162/089976699300016115

- Keysers C; Perrett DI (2004). "Demystifying social cognition: a Hebbian perspective". Trends in Cognitive Sciences. 8 (11): 501–507. PMID 15491904. doi:10.1016/j.tics.2004.09.005

Permissions

Index